# Life
# Before Birth

## REFLECTIONS ON THE EMBRYO DEBATE

# Life
# Before Birth

REFLECTIONS ON THE EMBRYO DEBATE

## Robert Edwards

Hutchinson
London Sydney Auckland Johannesburg

This edition first published in Great Britain
by Hutchinson, an imprint of Century Hutchinson
Ltd, Brookmount House, 62–65 Chandos Place,
London WC2N 4NW

Century Hutchinson Australia Pty Ltd,
89–91 Albion Street, Surry Hills, NSW 2010

Century Hutchinson New Zealand Ltd
PO Box 40–086, Glenfield, Auckland 10, New Zealand

Century Hutchinson South Africa (Pty) Ltd
PO Box 337, Bergvlei, 2012 South Africa

British Library Cataloguing in Publication Data

Edwards, R.G.
  Life before birth : reflections on the
  embryo debate.
  1. Embryology, Human—Research
  I. Title
  612'.64'0072    QM601

  ISBN 0-09-168150-2

Typeset in Monophoto Palatino by
Vision Typesetting, Manchester
Printed and bound in Great Britain by
Courier International Ltd, Tiptree, Essex

# Contents

*To Ruth*

# Acknowledgments

I wish to give my deepest thanks to my secretaries, Caroline Dawkin, Annabel Ward and especially Beverley Watts for their constant help and toleration of my frequent changes of text during the preparation of this book. I would also like to thank my Editor, David Compton, for his help and guidance, and Sue Avery, Mike Ashwood-Smith, Bridgett Masson, Alan Dexter and Edward Perrott for their most helpful comments on large sections of the draft. Finally, I am deeply indebted to those who kindly gave their permission for my use of their cartoons.

R.G. Edwards
26 April 1989

# Illustration Credits

The author and publishers would like to thank the following for permission to reproduce photographs and cartoons: Dr Tim Appleton; Granada Television; Peter Hollands; Brynmor Jones Library, University of Hull; Mail Newspapers; Oldham *Evening Chronicle*; Enoch Powell MBE; Rigby, Sun Newspapers; Gerald Scarfe; Syndication International; the Baroness Warnock.

# Foreword

Even as recently as the nineteen-thirties, when I was growing up with my two brothers in Manchester and going to high school there, the details of human conception and reproduction were largely a scientific mystery, an inaccessible series of poorly understood events that took place deep in a mother's womb. Nature decided when and how a baby would be conceived, when and with what genetic inheritance for good or ill it would be born, and when a woman would instead find herself sterile. Nature decided, usually for the best, and doctors stood by, smiling wisely. New diagnostic techniques were desperately needed, new family planning methods, and new ways to help the childless, but few were forthcoming.

Presumably, with my scientific bent, I was aware of all these needs by the time I reached university age, won the necessary scholarship, and had to decide upon a course of study — and certainly genetics and fertilisation interested me. But a far more powerful interest lingered from a period I had spent at the very beginning of the war as an evacuee on a hill farm in northern England, and I opted for agriculture at Bangor University instead, with a course in zoology thrown in for good measure. This proved a mistake. The scientist in me simply wasn't satisfied by the nature of the course taught at Bangor: after a four-year interruption for army service in the Near East, I bungled my finals and gained a muddled and less than distinguished degree.

But at that point fortune suddenly smiled on me. A studentship fell vacant in the Institute of Animal Genetics at Edinburgh University. I applied, and miraculously was accepted. This established the future direction of my scientific career and I became deeply involved in embryology, initially in that of the mouse and especially in its genetic control, and later in human embryology. I was fortunate also to come under the influence of Professor Waddington, who was not only an internationally respected embryological geneticist but also a man of profound moral integrity, a keen debater of ethical questions and the moral values of contemporary society.

These two disciplines, scientific and ethical, have guided me ever since. Most recently they have led me to write this book. Today many mysteries of human conception and reproduction have been solved. A scientific revolution is under way that has already brought enormous changes in man's understanding of himself, and that promises more and at an ever faster rate. As biology overlaps medicine more and more intimately, all aspects of our beginnings, of our growth and development from microscopic egg to mature adult, are under constant and intensive study. Female contraception, test-tube babies, genetic engineering, spare-part surgery . . . all these developments, unimaginable fifty years ago, already offer cures for many of our ills or repairs for many of our deficiencies. And the further this scientific revolution permeates medicine and other areas such as animal husbandry, the more deeply it challenges our ethical judgments, even our most fundamental beliefs.

This is the point at which the new biology meets not only ethics, religion and philosophy, but also politics, law and organised society. For many of these scientific developments put into question traditional social customs and assumptions. Research into the first stages of embryonic life, into the genetic make-up of an embryo, into the gradual emergence of organs as embryo becomes fetus and then child, all this has taught us how to conceive human beings in-vitro in the laboratory, how to insert new genes into animal embryos, even how to bring together successfully the eggs and spermatozoa of couples separated by great distances, even by death itself. Thus even traditional notions of parentage are made obsolete and, as further advances are promised, decisions must be taken – political decisions, legal decisions, personal decisions – as to whether such techniques are permissible, and if so then to what if any degree they should be controlled.

Today we have reached a stage when each new scientific advance confusingly raises both the hopes and the fears of ordinary men and women: should it be welcomed as a godsend, a lasting benefit to us all, or should it be rejected as a divisive force, a threat to ancient and reassuring beliefs? Even those scientists and clinicians who know best the strengths and weaknesses of each new development are anxious and troubled as they look ahead, for they are only too aware that today's remote possibility can become – and at a pace far quicker than any accompanying social adjustment – tomorrow's standard practice.

This book is intended to provide a frank account of one such field of study, the science of embryology and its many applications (of which the creation of test-tube babies is perhaps the best known), together with its implications for humanity, the ethical questions it raises and the political and legal decisions it makes necessary. My credentials for writing are simple. In human terms, I am fortunate enough to be long and very happily married, with five daughters (and several dogs), and we live on a small farm just outside Cambridge. In political terms, I served for five years as a Labour member of the Cambridge City Council and remain deeply interested in the way in which Britain is governed. In professional terms, I travel widely as a scientist, giving lectures and attending seminars, I run an internationally known fertility clinic, and since 1985 I have been Professor of Human Reproduction at Cambridge University.

The major theme of my book is the progress made over

the last twelve years in in-vitro fertilisation as a technique for overcoming human infertility, but I also deal with its wider implications in the fields of genetic engineering, of the alleviation of inherited disease, of spare-part surgery using animal or human embryonic cell tissue, and also with such novel means of parentage as embryo donation and surrogate motherhood.

I myself helped to pioneer many of these developments, and inevitably have had to face the many moral dilemmas they present, and I hope that I have not shrunk here from open debate or uncompromising judgments. It may well be that an understanding of the ethics involved in this field is of even greater importance to society than the scientific breakthroughs themselves; but in any case the future of scientific and medical research would be seriously endangered if there were any public suspicion of an Establishment cover-up. Such new and radical departures are of such fundamental importance to humanity that total openness is essential. The rights and wrongs *must* be discussed. Today, in the nineteen-eighties, bio-ethics — or moral philosophy in biology, or whatever label is used — have irrevocably entered the public domain. They are part of the embryo debate to which all of us, men and women, scientists and politicians, clerics and laity, doctors, lawyers and philosophers, have our own contribution to make. It's a debate that needs facts as well as frankness, and I hope this book provides both.

# 1
# Going it alone

1978. It's not really very long ago, but it seems so to me. Those last anxious weeks of waiting, in July 1978, for the birth of Mr and Mrs John Brown's baby seem like another lifetime, another world. We waited, the Browns and our tiny medical team, Jean, Patrick and I, counting the days and biting our nails. And the press waited too, cluttering the hospital corridors, virtually camping in the grounds, for word had got out about this very special pregnancy and each reporter was determined to be first with the exciting news and pictures.

Today, in-vitro fertilisation is a medical commonplace, widely practised, and I and scientists like me travel the world advising, lecturing, and attending seminars. But back in 1978 Jean and Patrick and I were working virtually on our own. Very few people, hardly any in the British medical establishment, took seriously our dream of bringing hope to the large number of couples – over four thousand newly-weds each year in Britain alone – who suffer from problems of infertility.

Patrick Steptoe was the physician in our team, a consultant gynaecologist of immense warmth, experience and authority. I was the research scientist, the nuts-and-bolts man, and Jean Purdy was our laboratory assistant. Indeed, she was far more than that, for she had once been a nurse and she was now a good friend and collaborator.

As for myself, all my professional life the wonders and

mysteries of early embryonic life had fascinated me and filled me with awe. Human infertility, too, had long concerned me. A family man myself, I was moved by the very real distress of childless couples I knew. And so it was that, when an intriguing possibility emerged from my research work on mice, first in Edinburgh and then in Cambridge, I followed it up eagerly. Such childless couples might just be helped to have their own children by means of a process known as in-vitro fertilisation – that is, the fertilisation of a woman's egg by her husband's sperm in a culture dish outside her body and the return of that fertilised egg to her womb, to be nurtured there for an otherwise perfectly normal pregnancy.

Nobody can create human life artificially, not in a test-tube, a Petri dish, or anywhere else. Such claims are ridiculous, pathetically arrogant. Life is uniquely *there*, bursting out everywhere, a wonderful part of our universe. The most that any of us can do is to help to make life possible, and to make it healthy and good. And that was what I wanted to do – to help to make human life possible, and healthy, and good.

And now, in July 1978, all the preliminary work was over. Our little team in the Oldham and General District Hospital had done all it could. Mrs Brown, previously unable to conceive, was nine months pregnant. All the signs were good. Only the waiting remained, for Nature to take its course.

On 25 July 1978, Louise Brown was born. She was a lovely baby, 5 lb 12 oz, and her parents' joy was our joy. It was an emotional occasion. Patrick had performed the delivery by Caesarian section. Inside the operating theatre, I waited for my turn to hold Louise in my arms and to marvel – as always with a new baby – at her tiny wrinkled perfection. There was laughter and there were happy tears.

Meanwhile hundreds of eager pressmen were sending their stories round the world. For the first time a child had been conceived in vitro and then successfully returned to

GG 705097

1 & 2 ELIZ. 2 CH. 20

**CERTIFICATE** **OF BIRTH**

Name and Surname Louise Joy BROWN

Sex Female

Date of Birth Twenty Fifth July 1978

Place ( Registration
of ( District Oldham

Birth ( Sub-district Boundary Park

I, JOAN BAMFORD Registrar of Births and Deaths
for the sub-district of BOUNDARY PARK in the
Registration District of OLDHAM do hereby
certify that the above particulars have been compiled from an entry in
a register in my custody.

Date - 3 AUG 1978

YPAOT25

Registrar of Births and Deaths.

CAUTION:—*Any person who (1) falsifies any of the particulars on this certificate, or
(2) uses a falsified certificate as true, knowing it to be false, is liable to prosecution.*

grow in its mother's womb. It was a message of hope to
countless unhappily childless couples. It was also the first
step for Jean and Patrick and me on a long journey, long and
rewarding but often contentious and difficult.

Louise Brown's birth was a media sensation. As she slept
peacefully in her cot her every detail was flashed excitedly
from country to country. There were pictures galore,
congratulations for her parents and us, admiration for her.

'Baby of the century,' was how the *Daily Express* saw her
(11 July 1978).

'The lovely Louise,' announced the *Daily Mail* (27 July
1978).

'Their No. 1 girl is just perfect!' claimed the local Oldham
paper, the *Chronicle*, (29 July 1978).

But storm clouds were already gathering. We decided to overlook them at the time, living in a busy, happy, uncomplicated daze, but they were to loom over us ever more thickly as the years went by, just as they had done in the years before Louise's birth.

'The test-tube baby debate begins; grievous sin or precious gift?' (*Philadelphia Inquirer*, 29 July 1978)

'Mixed blessings.' (*New York Times*, 30 July 1978)

The underlying fears, of course, were of future morally complex developments, of genetic engineering, of impermissible research upon the unborn, of the possibilities for surrogate motherhood, for the storing of frozen embryos, for the ability to choose a baby's sex. These were real fears, and reasonable too, for medical science was moving into an area for which it had as yet very few moral or ethical criteria. They were only tentatively voiced to begin with, and for a while they were drowned out by the wonder and sheer excitement of Louise's birth. Happy stories dominated the news. Lesley and John Brown had their daughter, and now they were taking her home to Bristol. The world had greeted its first test-tube baby. Ethical arguments could wait.

Even so, it had to be admitted that conceiving children outside the mother was a novel idea. So novel, in fact, that until that July very few people had thought it possible — except Jean and Patrick and myself, working away in isolation in Oldham. And even now many doctors and gynaecologists were refusing to believe us, claiming that Louise had been conceived in the usual manner, and that in-vitro fertilisation was all a trick.

It was hard to blame them. Our present success had been the result of a long uphill struggle — twenty years and more since my interest in infertility had first been roused during my work as a young postgraduate student in Edinburgh University, working under the distinguished embryologists and geneticists Professor Waddington and Alan Beatty, dosing female mice with fertility drugs in order to produce sufficient mouse embryos for my doctoral research work. Problems of mouse fertility were quickly solved – but when I left Edinburgh and wished to extend my work to include human embryos, the path was fraught with far greater difficulties.

The main snag proved to be a scarcity of research materials: in this case, human eggs. For several years my only source of these was pieces of ovary excised for clinical reasons by gynaecologists sympathetic enough to my work to be willing to collaborate by passing them on to me. Such people, perhaps unsurprisingly, were hard to find.

My curiosity was wide-ranging. Because they seemed so important to me, I was fired with an ambition to study the beginnings of human life, to uncover the fundamental secrets of fertilisation and the earliest stages of embryonic development. I wanted to find out more about human chromosomes, and why some babies were born with one too many, such as those with Down's syndrome. I wanted to study the hormones of reproduction and contraception. I wanted to observe in minute detail how two, four, eight and more cells form in the embryo. And I wanted to find a remedy for some forms of human infertility.

Such interests lie where science meets medicine and both have to satisfy society. The ethical questions they raise had always concerned me. They concerned others too, clerics, ethicists, politicians, reporters – professionals who filled me with awe and foreboding in those early, uncertain days, just as they do many of my young contemporaries now. Research results could so easily be misunderstood; muddled or dire conclusions could so easily be drawn. Even so, I was determined to press ahead with my ideas. There were thousands of desperate patients in urgent need of the hope they offered.

Most gynaecologists turned away in blank disbelief when I tried to explain my intentions. Who was this young scientist with his harebrained schemes? In those days fertilised human eggs and embryos had hardly ever been seen outside the human body and here was I, not even a medical doctor, proposing to produce them in a culture dish! I toured the world, when my work would let me, in search of human eggs. Mostly the response was the same – disbelief sometimes mixed with outrage. But fortunately just enough were friendly, especially two gynaecologists in London, Molly Rose and Victor Lewis, and two in the USA, Howard Jones and Bob McGaughey. They collaborated directly and helped me through the difficult beginnings, providing vital pieces of ovary until eventually, in 1964, with perseverance and a lot of luck, I got the conditions right and human eggs ripened in my culture dishes just as mouse eggs had done.

'Births may be by proxy,' commented a reporter in the *Sunday Times* on 7 November 1965, after my first report on ripening human eggs had appeared in the *Lancet*.

He was probably the first newsman to see the future clearly.

'Culture of early human embryos is imminent,' announced *World Medicine* in December that year, sticking to the facts and soberly refusing to speculate.

And even *World Medicine*'s 'imminent' was to prove optimistic. Always handicapped by shortages of research materials, I met delays and obstacles at every turn. Until, in 1968, I met Patrick Steptoe.

I had read in a Cambridge library of his laparoscopy work. It was a technique for passing fibre-optical tubes into the abdominal cavity, to examine its organs and to direct the excision of pieces of tissue by remote control. I rang him first. Then we met after a seminar. Could he reach the ovary, I asked him, and collect eggs from there without distressing the patient? He said he was sure he could – moreover, he liked the sound of my work and was willing to help. His laparoscopy promised me an uncomplicated, almost unlimited supply of exactly the eggs I needed, so we joined forces.

Unfortunately for me, Patrick was a senior consultant

gynaecologist up in Oldham, Lancashire, with a Regional Health Authority that gave him the fullest possible support, while I was now firmly settled with my wife and family in Cambridge, lecturing and carrying out my research. This geographical separation was to lead to ten years of frequent 200-mile car journeys for me and one or other of my research technicians, from a Cambridge lecture hall to an Oldham operating theatre and back again. We often tried to break the pattern by arranging a move for one of us, but nothing ever came of it. The phone would ring in Cambridge — Patrick was performing a laparoscopy that afternoon and would have eggs for me by four o'clock — and out my technician and I would rush to the car, for the eggs had to be absolutely fresh if we were to have any hope of fertilising them.

Of all my technicians, Jean was the most determined and loyal, and we three were soon doing all the work together. Progress was encouraging. In many ways it was a repeat of my work with mice back in Edinburgh: we would administer fertility drugs, in this case to the wife of an infertile couple, then pluck fresh ripening eggs from her ovary exactly on time. Her eggs would then be fertilised with her husband's spermatozoa, and their embryos grew in our culture dishes. The next stage was more difficult, replacing one or two of these embryos via her vagina into her womb, just as I had dreamed of years before, and bringing about a pregnancy . . . But the fertility drugs were wonderful, providing a windfall of eggs, six, seven, occasionally even more from a patient. Fertilisation in vitro was conquered, and embryos grew beautifully in our culture dishes. Sooner or later we were bound to succeed in implanting them.

Our patients were magnificent, returning repeatedly for tests and examinations, sustained by their hopes for a child at long last, after every other treatment had failed. We for our part remained guardedly optimistic, while the press — which followed our every move — was always on the look-out for sensation. In fact the newspapers exactly reflected society's conflicting emotions, its hopes and fears, and its ill-informed opinions.

'Test-tube life outside the body,' the *Daily Express* correctly reported on 14 February 1969 – only to elaborate, just one day later, 'Row flares over test-tube babies.'

The public debate between science and ethics had ignited, and has burned brightly ever since.

'Tube babies "Far off".' (The *Guardian*, 15 February 1969)

'Views on experiment divided.' (*The Times*, 15 February 1969)

'Ban the test-tube baby.' The *Sun*, 25 February 1970)

'Test-tube baby "murder" attacked by Dr Heenan.' (The *Daily Telegraph*, February 1969)

'Chief Rabbi slams test-tube stud farming' (The *Sunday Express*, 1 March 1970)

'The obsolescent mother.' (*Atlantic Monthly*, May 1971)

But right at the beginning, in February 1969, *The Times* had summed up the issues well: 'It is the implications rather than the direct consequences of the first successful fertilis-ation of a human egg in a test-tube that pose the most searching moral problems.'

With that, Jean and Patrick and I were in complete agreement. But we had more than ethical problems to cope with: in spite of an excellent supply of beautifully fertilised eggs, pregnancies were proving hard to come by. It took five years of perseverance, of tests and observation and minute changes in technical procedure, before, in 1975, an undoubted fetus was achieved. We were elated as it grew in its mother for twelve weeks. But then, very sadly, it was found to be ectopic – that is, implanted in its mother's Fallopian tubes rather than in her womb – and it threatened her life, and so had to be removed.

We reported this episode in the *Lancet*: 'A human embryo in transition between morula and blastocyst after culture in-vitro was reintroduced into the mother's uterus via the cervix. The resulting embryo was . . . located in the oviduct. It was removed at thirteen weeks of gestation.'

I vividly remember our disappointment. But I also remember that mother. When she left the hospital with her husband the two of them stopped and turned to Patrick. 'Can we try again, doctor?' her husband asked.

Patrick nodded. Of course they could try again. And of course, with such a poignant demonstration of need and of faith in us, we too would try again. And again and again.

Who was following our lead? The advantages all lay elsewhere in large departments of obstetrics and gynaecology, not with our minute team. An Australian effort failed following unbelievably fanciful claims of a very short-lived pregnancy. One American tried for several years, another achieved fertilisation before succumbing to ethical objections while another – trained by us – hesitated back home until the whole world was doing IVF. An Italian claimed to be growing human fetuses in bottles for weeks on end, a Briton claimed he'd had test-tube babies everywhere which couldn't be found, and another Briton, also trained by us, tried hard without success. We were still alone, confident now after that ectopic pregnancy.

The problem seemed to lie with the fertility drugs. Although necessary in order to guarantee an adequate supply of eggs, they distorted the mother's hormonal balance so that pregnancy became virtually impossible. Many lines of research lay open to us, but time was running out – Patrick's retirement from the National Health Service was fast approaching. With new urgency we tried other techniques, placing spermatozoa in a wife's oviducts just before she ovulated, freezing her eggs and embryos and then thawing them for replacement later, after the effects of the fertility drugs had worn off. We tried different drugs too, in different dosages, and over different periods of time. But success still eluded us.

Finally, as Patrick's retirement came very close, we abandoned the use of drugs altogether and returned to the natural menstrual cycle. With infinite care he plucked one single ripening egg from the one growing follicle. Fertilisation took place safely and successfully in the culture medium. The embryo developed into eight cells. We replaced it in its mother . . .

This is how Louise Brown was conceived. And when we heard her vigorous crying a moment or so after delivery, every single day of our ten long years of penny-pinching struggle was rewarded. Every mile driven, every hour of sleep lost, every disappointment, every unjust criticism — they had all been worth it. The baby Louise was safe in her mother's arms: what an answer to our accusers, especially the Vatican Press Officer who had branded our work as 'immoral . . . and absolutely illicit'.

Our financial troubles, we thought, were over. Up to then we had worked on a shoestring, our resources pathetically meagre. The Oldham Health Authority, with rare courage and vision, had done its best for us, but its funds inevitably were strictly limited: there had been virtually no money for new equipment, or sophisticated chemicals, or even the endless travel. Outside appeals within the British Establishment were useless. The President of the Royal College of Obstetricians and Gynaecologists, Sir John Peel, offered to help but nothing came of it: he gave no reasons but presumably he thought we were wasting our time. The British Medical Research Council also refused us: they argued that laparoscopy was dangerous and insisted that experiments be carried out on rhesus monkeys first. Yet Patrick was a world authority on laparoscopy, which carried minimum dangers to patients, and the monkeys had such distinctive ovaries and convoluted reproductive tracts that research carried out on them had little or no application to humans.

For a while the American Ford Foundation gave generously — I was enormously grateful, but even so it was ironic for me, a committed British socialist, to have to turn to foreign capitalists for funds — but they pulled out in the mid-seventies, worried by the ethical controversy surrounding in-vitro fertilisation in the USA. It was in fact a few individuals who kept us going, especially an American benefactress who helped when we needed it most. Bless them, for they made our work possible.

Now, however, all that was surely over. Within a very short time two more babies conceived in vitro were born, one sadly premature, demonstrating the practicality of this new method of human conception. The novelty was wearing off. All the initial shock resulting from the establishment of human life for the first time outside the human body – a shattering concept to many people – was over. The time had come for a large medical research centre and clinic in which to carry on and develop our work, and preferably in Cambridge, my university.

We made our plans. Two happy, healthy test-tube babies were surely enough to win us widespread support. A major institute in Cambridge was needed, with premises, staff and equipment – and even a place for Patrick, who had now retired from the National Health Service. And with the results we could show there should be no problems. Sophisticated institutes in science and medicine had often been founded on far less. Part-time in-vitro fertilisation and research was over: it was a full-time job now. Things had to change.

I sounded out the Cambridge authorities. There were compliments, and praise for the work we'd done, and guarded offers of premises and funding. I took them at their word – I wasn't worried, bureaucracies were always cautious – and we began packing up in Oldham.

Only Jean was doubtful.

'Why not carry on here while we can, while we're successful?' she asked, even as we were stacking our equipment ready for the journey to Cambridge. 'Everything's organised here, the staff know what to do, and our methods are working. Why change now? We were never able to get proper support in Cambridge before – why take the risk now?'

I ignored her plea. It was too late anyway – plans were

multiplying in my head: controlled environment laboratories, specialist staff, sunny wards filled with happy
pregnant women. The bit was between my teeth.

When we reached Cambridge, however, the reality was
rather less appealing. The authorities seemed to have no
conception of the facilities we would need. My fault, for not
properly explaining? Theirs, for not listening? I don't know.
But instead of a large, fully-serviced clinic with operating
theatres, patient beds, and a supporting staff to cope with a
heavy schedule of operations, we were offered two rooms
in old Addenbrooke's Hospital: an ancient operating theatre
up on the third floor, and a shed on the ground floor for our
laboratory. Eggs collected from patients upstairs would
have to be taken downstairs for fertilisation, and embryos
would have to be carried back upstairs again for replacement in their mothers. Upstairs, downstairs with such
delicate and precious cargo, seven or eight times a day –
that was worse than in Oldham, where at least the
laboratory and operating theatre were next to each other.

Suddenly we were homeless. We couldn't return to
Oldham – others were already using our accommodation –
and the facilities offered in Cambridge simply were not
practicable. Government, in the form of the Department of
Health, remained woodenly uninterested. There was only
one other possibility: at one time, rather unusually, the
Editor of the *Daily Mail* had promised help if we really
needed it.

We really needed it. Was he still interested? He was, and
so was his parent company. So much so that they asked us
to search for premises suitable for a private clinic.

A private clinic! I had never contemplated such a
possibility, even in my wildest dreams. A private clinic –
millions of pounds of investment! Not to mention the
further blow to my socialist conscience. And anyway, a
clinic outside the National Health Service sounded quite
impossible. But even the impossible became acceptable as
time passed, and nothing else was offered, and our need

grew ever more acute. Finally we accepted that if we were
to continue our work at all, a private clinic was our only
chance.

It was an enterprise that would quickly be copied
worldwide. Private clinics for in-vitro fertilisation would
mushroom, and private fortunes would be made. But we
worried about none of this, of course, as we started our
search for suitable premises. It was that, or give up
altogether.

I had started to write a textbook (*Conception in the Human
Female*, Academic Press, London, 1980), exploring every
aspect of female reproduction. I was living at home in
Cambridge and working hard, and Patrick was still based
miles away, up at his house in Rochdale. It was poor Jean,
therefore, living close by me in Cambridge, who was
available to tramp round the estate agents.

'Off you go,' I told her, 'and don't come back till you've
found a suitable house for our clinic. A pleasant place, where
patients can stay comfortably, not cramped but close
enough for them to help each other as they did up in
Oldham. And of course, not too far from Cambridge.'

Loyally she set off, full of hope, to return glumly at the
end of several days.

'No luck,' she reported. 'I've seen large houses, mansions,
ancient monuments, disused factories, derelict schools, all
sorts . . . but nothing remotely like what we need.'

'Well, try again tomorrow,' I insisted, going anxiously
back to my textbook. The publishers were already harrying
me.

This time Jean returned with photographs and a
brochure.

'I've seen the most marvellous place!' she exclaimed. 'It's
fabulous, beautiful, everything I've always dreamed of.' She
showed me an aerial photograph. 'It's called Bourn Hall. It's
practically a stately home. It's over four hundred years old,
and it stands in its own park.'

I stared at the picture. It showed a small, beautifully

proportioned manor house in mellow red brick, with superb roofs and chimneys, set in lovely parkland. It would make a wonderful clinic, it would make a wonderful anything . . . and the brochure said it was only about eight miles from Cambridge. But surely it was too grand for us, too expensive to contemplate? Houses like that were used for hotels, country clubs, rich men's leisure centres.

'There are roughly eight bedrooms,' Jean told me, watching me warily out of the corner of her eye. 'The downstairs rooms are fine for us, and there are some very useful outbuildings. It's in a good state of repair, but the agent says the services need some attention. It'd be ideal for us.' She paused. 'The price is £250,000.'

A quarter of a million pounds. Where on earth would money like that come from? It was far beyond any sum I had ever contemplated. And the purchase price was only the beginning. Laying drains and supplying electricity to the standards of a properly licensed clinic are expensive items. Conversions would be needed, furnishing and decoration, and then the medical and scientific equipment: a high-tech laboratory with purified air and specialised refrigeration . . . not to mention the salaries for doctors, nurses, embryologists. The list of expenses was never-ending. Even so, Patrick was sent for and we went to have a look. We had to.

Bourn Hall turned out to be a beautiful Jacobean building, with exquisite period windows and detailing in the brickwork, its own stables and outbuildings, even its own little chapel, and set in a park of some twenty acres. It was surrounded by an ancient moat and its motto, carved above the door, was *'Jour de ma vie'* − which is probably best translated as *'My every day is a whole life'* − inherited from its very first Huguenot owner, which seemed particularly suitable for our future patients.

But a quarter of a million pounds was still an awful lot of money, so Jean continued her search, looking for a less expensive alternative. She found all sorts, country houses that were too small, country houses that were too big, country houses that were too far away, even an ancient bedraggled university department. None was suitable. Only Bourn Hall, still on the market, filled our requirements.

Tentatively we approached the Editor of the *Daily Mail* again. Amazingly his company acted without hesitation, buying the Hall and immediately appointing an architect, skilled staff, accountants, surveyors and engineers. They worked with wonderful speed. The grounds were surveyed, an outline plan was made, and within a very few weeks we were passionately debating our detailed specifications for the new clinic. Temporary cabins were built in the grounds to serve for six months while the main building was being converted, and we hoped to be accepting our first patients by the end of April – only nine months after Louise's birth.

The blow fell in early April 1979. On the strength of a single phone call all work at Bourn Hall was stopped and our friends pulled out. I never discovered their reason. Someone told us they'd taken fright because, should an abnormal baby be born at a planned associated clinic in the United States, they would risk a court action there and the confiscation of their American holdings. But in any case our hopes went with them, for there was now no money. The workers departed, the new temporary cabins stood desolated, empty, and Bourn Hall returned to silence and peaceful decay.

Weeks and months passed. Our *Daily Mail* backers were kind to us. They held the Hall on our behalf and, to help us raise money so that we could buy it ourselves, they introduced us to a financier, Alan Dexter, an expert in our sort of problem. We would have to go it alone, just as in Oldham, and Alan began his search for finance, holding meeting after meeting, including one in a deserted Bourn Hall in the depths of 1979's bitter winter, with no heating at all in its echoing rooms and passages. I watched in dismay as my colleagues' noses turned slowly blue with the cold and was hardly surprised when, on that day at least, no windfall of millions was produced.

It was at about this time, early in 1980, that a group of Australian doctors in Melbourne announced the first antipodean test-tube baby. They'd had enormous difficulties and still seemed despondent and doubtful about the potential of IVF. They were our first followers; we'd personally told them all we knew a year or so earlier.

'Australia's first test-tube baby . . . the result of an eight-year, $A1.2m programme involving forty Melbourne specialists,' *The Times* reported in February 1980. $A1.2m came to roughly half a million pounds — I only wished we ourselves had that sort of money!

In fact Alan was facing rebuff after rebuff. As he was to write later in the *Medical News*, 'Incredible as it seems . . . there were millions of dollars amassed in the States to back such a clinic, but no one knew how to do it . . . Here, where the technique had been perfected, there was no interest.'

Miraculously, he was eventually able to sort our problems out, raising funds from a financial company, ICFC. By conserving our limited resources and abandoning most of the work on the house itself, the Bourn Hall clinic was opened in October 1980, its five temporary cabins serving as wards, operating theatre and embryology laboratory. We were still on a shoestring and the Minister of Health — as slow to accept new ideas as ever — still declined to help us.

'Just over two years after Louise Brown . . . was born, Cambridge physiologist Professor Robert Edwards, and gynaecologist Mr Patrick Steptoe . . . have opened their own clinic,' the *Medical News* reported on 9 October 1980. 'The clinic opened quietly enough by admitting eleven patients . . . The clinic is no spectacle of private hospital luxury.'

But times for us were very different from the Oldham days. Oldham had stood for original research, every step exciting and new, as almost every method still in use today was pioneered. Now, as the first pregnancies were established, we were permanently committed, well into the future, with our main concern to keep standards consistent and high over the years to come.

The first Bourn Hall baby was born in 1981. We ran up a flag on the flagpole to salute it, the first of many.

'Five new test-tube babies and sixty more on the way,' *The Times* reported on 6 October 1981, one year after Bourn Hall had opened.

The wasted two years since Louise's birth were forgotten. There had been further developments in Australia where a biologist, Alan Trounson, had joined the team to buck them up; he had first finished a period of research in Cambridge. They, and a team led by Howard Jones in the USA, were moving after reintroducing the fertility drugs we had used in Oldham. But we were leaving the rest of the world behind in numbers of pregnancies. Curious visiting experts increased in numbers, cramming our tiny temporary laboratories as they noted every detail of every procedure. We were part of Britain's export drive too — babies conceived in Bourn Hall were the first conceived in-vitro to be born in the USA, Canada, Greece, Yugoslavia and many other countries.

At Bourn Hall we kept our costs to the patient as low as was humanly possible. We were lucky too — our backers weren't greedy. But we watched sadly as more and more doctors sized up their prospects and did their calculations. Many were altruistic. Others were outspokenly mercenary, planning to plunder the endless queues of childless, hopeful patients, totting up the pay beds to be filled. Most of these doctors passed through Bourn Hall, accepting our free advice as they planned chains of clinics like Woolworths across a country or continent. Some repaid us by trying to entice our staff away with huge salaries and fabulous opportunities in exotic countries.

Clearly conception in vitro was going to be slow in its spread to the poorer sections of society. The British National Health Service remained unconvinced. It must have been bitter for the infertile to have paid their state dues yet now to be excluded from the treatment they most desired. Medical science offered them this glimpse of happiness, yet if they wanted a family, a stake in the future, they'd have to pay for it.

For a while things improved. Ian Craft started a public IVF service at the Royal Free Hospital in London, and a similar initiative was begun in Manchester. The press gave them banner headlines:

'Rush for test-tube babies as twins are born on NHS.' (The *Daily Telegraph*, 1 May 1982)

'Test-tube babies make NHS proud.' (*The Times*, 9 July 1983)

One by one, however, these public health projects collapsed. Ian Craft was obliged to move to the private Cromwell Hospital, and others of his colleagues went partly or completely that way. Penelope Leach wrote the quote of the week in 1986:

'You can't have IVF unless you are rich.' (The *Guardian*, 24 April 1986)

Fresh ideas were coming from all over the world. A Scandinavian group was able to replace laparoscopy with ultrasound, guiding needles through the abdomen and into the ovary as if by radar, avoiding the need for general anaesthesia. Then ultrasound became even simpler, as needles were passed through the vaginal wall itself to collect the eggs – since the two ovaries lie close to the vagina they could now be reached without any harm. Advances we had dreamed of in Oldham were slowly coming true.

Scientists in Australia, Holland and France were now freezing human embryos, just as we had done in Oldham and later at Bourn Hall. It was a controversial step, and so was the occluding of damaged Fallopian tubes, which Patrick sometimes did to avoid ectopic pregnancies. Then a breakthrough came for those patients with no obvious cause of infertility, as unfertilised eggs were placed together with spermatozoa in the wife's healthy tubes, and pregnancies began.

'Pregnancy after translaparoscopic gamete intrafallopian transfer,' was the tongue-twisting title of the piece in the *Lancet* by its Argentinian inventor, Ricardo Asch, and his colleagues.

He called the procedure itself GIFT, a lovely name, and he succeeded where we had earlier failed. Simpler still, spermatozoa were injected into the wife's abdominal cavity after she had ovulated, to be drawn into her oviduct by its own powerful currents. The French inventors called this DIPI, for 'direct intraperitoneal insemination'. Eggs and spermatozoa were even successfully injected together into the abdomen to result in pregnancies.

In 1985 the number of Bourn Hall pregnancies passed one thousand – more than in the whole of the USA or in Australia and New Zealand combined, and each one conceived in our 'temporary' cabins, still going strong. The first Russian IVF baby was shown on Moscow television in 1986, and in the same year the first IVF baby was conceived and born in Bombay.

More clinics opened. In Australia a working clinic was bought by Americans and transported, its doctors, scientists, equipment, lock stock and barrel, to Los Angeles. By 1986 there were more than forty clinics each in Britain, France and Germany, fourteen in Australia, a hundred and fifty in the USA. Conception in vitro spread to China, the Middle East, Colombia and Zimbabwe.

'First test-tube baby under way in Black Africa,' claimed a 1987 headline in *The Times*, going on to quote a gynaecologist in Zimbabwe: 'Even before the official announcement . . . requests had come in from couples in neighbouring Botswana and Zambia . . . We expect to be swamped.'

These remarks prompted a typically carping editorial comment: 'The development appears strange in a country with a population growth rate put at 3.2 per cent per annum . . . The reason lies in the southern African system of *roora* or bride price . . . which will not be handed over until after the wife falls pregnant.'

Was this really why couples wanted IVF in Zimbabwe? If so, then why were they so different from the other couples all over the world who also wanted test-tube babies? Why were they so different from couples in the USA, for example, who were so desperate that they were willing to pay surrogate mothers to carry their babies for them, if they couldn't gestate their own?

Not that such ill-informed comments were anything new. They were the less worthy part of the storm of genuine ethical concern that was sweeping the world. Those first 1978 rumblings of disquiet had grown to a positive thunder, as statesmen and parliaments, philosophers and priests of every possible persuasion, came to grips with the moral issues involved in conceiving babies in vitro, in surrogate motherhood, in research on living embryos, in the freezing of embryos or the donation of eggs, sperm or embryos from one person to another. Commissions and official boards of inquiry were established. The Warnock Committee in Britain and the Waller Committee in Australia were government appointed, and soon to be matched by other countries in Western Europe. Watchdog organisations were formed, including a Voluntary Licensing Authority in Britain and a National Ethical Committee in France.

And still the wonder of that birth persisted, even until Louise's tenth birthday: 'For this was not just the birth of a five-pound baby girl with a thatch of blond hair and healthy appetite; it was a watershed in human evolution, one of the twentieth century's most important events, suddenly every bit as remarkable as man's first steps on the moon and the splitting of the atom,' wrote Michael Pirrie in the *Melbourne Age*, 25 July 1988. Some newspapers even recognised its importance in their birthday's column, usually filled with

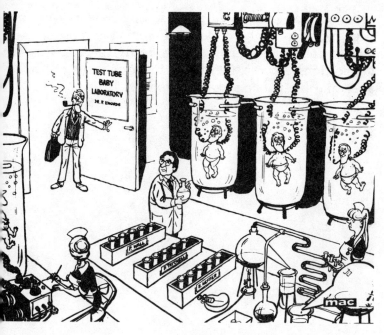

'Okay Edwards — The B.M.A. have lifted their ban — Now for Heaven's sake, get a move on!'

generals and admirals and ancient politicians, for the *Independent* finally decided that its list for 25 July should be headed by 'Louise Brown, 10'. As for Louise, she described herself: 'I am a test tube big girl now' (*Sunday Mirror*, 24 July 1988).

As the ethical controversy grew it began to engulf all scientific or medical considerations, ignoring objective truth in its fervour. It engulfed me too, as the arguments intensified and the abuse grew shriller — so much so that, although the most unlitigious of people, I became involved in libel actions in the High Court, seven of them eventually, against such opponents as *The Times* newspapers and the British Medical Association.

It all seemed a very long way from those mice back in the animal house at Edinburgh University. But the uncomfortable fact remained that the reproductive principles we had established in those tiny rodents had now been found to apply to men and women in most of their details, and none of us was quite ready to deal with the implications. And so, inevitably, the arguments had to be aired and the public properly informed.

# 2
# Why bother with infertility?

The first fact we must face is that many people are ambivalent in their attitudes towards in-vitro fertilisation as a treatment for human infertility. These are decent, caring people, and their concerns must be taken seriously. They may sympathise with their unhappily childless friends, and will rejoice with them if a baby is eventually born, but they often have vague secret reservations. They feel that simple therapies, such as diet, drugs, even minor surgery, are probably all right, but they worry about devoting expensive resources to complicated procedures for curing infertility when too many children are being born anyway. And what about the ethics of the research that has made in-vitro fertilisation possible? Is it right to tinker like this with the beginnings of human life? And besides, where's it all going to end?

More specific questions are raised by those critics who openly campaign for in-vitro fertilisation to be banned, and indeed all work on human embryos. There is something unacceptably intrusive, even immoral, they say, about growing human embryos in a dish. What happens to those that are not replaced in their mother? And what about those embryos that *are* replaced, only to be culled later when it's found that too many have successfully implanted? Wouldn't the scientists involved be better employed finding a cure for AIDS? Why can't infertile couples adopt unwanted babies and so avoid all these complex and dubious procedures? If there *aren't* enough unwanted babies to go round, why not deal with that by banning most abortions? And anyway, infertility isn't like cancer, or heart disease, or kidney failure. It's neither life-threatening nor does it preclude happiness. Lots of people who don't have any children get along perfectly well, so isn't there really something rather self-indulgent about all these couples who refuse to accept that they were simply never meant to be parents?

Arguments against in-vitro fertilisation chase off in so many different directions that I must begin by making clear exactly what the fuss is all about. In-vitro conception occurs when a ripe human egg is removed from a woman, fertilised by human sperm in a dish containing a nutrient solution, allowed to develop there until the resulting tiny embryo is clearly vigorous and normal, and then replaced in her womb. The intention is that it will grow there for the usual period of gestation and eventually be born as a perfectly normal, healthy baby. The woman and man concerned are usually in an established stable relationship, but not always. Occasionally they don't even know each other: the sperm can come from a donor, so can the egg, and so even can the womb that carries the child until its birth.

An egg in a dish, to which sperm is added . . . although apparently simple, IVF is in fact a very delicate procedure. Many tests are needed, over a lengthy period, and even so some factors outside our control still dictate whether or not a particular embryo will implant properly in the lining of a womb. This, after all, is the pattern in nature, where conception is by no means inevitable, even at the most favourable time in the woman's reproductive cycle. In IVF, to improve the chances of success, several embryos are usually prepared and replaced during any one treatment, but even so a woman may have to make repeated visits to the clinic before she becomes pregnant. Sadly, there are some women for whom the procedure is never successful.

So why are they willing to go through all this anxiety, inconvenience, discomfort, and heart-ache? Why do we doctors and scientists let them?

Clearly the cultural pressures on men and women to reproduce are enormous. 'There is a long-standing Christian concern that marriage, whenever possible, should lead to parenthood,' wrote a board set up by the Church of England to study the matter in 1985. On a secular level, too, the pressures are wide-ranging. Laws of inheritance, the continuance of family name and position, the perceived roles of women as mothers and men as providers, the extensions of identity that children provide, the sense of purpose given by their rearing, the pride in their successes, the hope of their companionship and support in their parents' old age, even the promise they bring of grandchildren – the social expectations fulfilled by children are many and powerful.

These have long been formalised in manifestos and documents, most significantly perhaps in Article 12 of the European Convention of Human Rights: 'Men and women of marriageable age have the right to marry and found a family according to the national laws governing the exercise of that right.'

There are pressures of custom, also: the community's broad assumption that childless couples are in some way diminished, failed, subjects for pity or even disapproval. And then, of course, there are economic pressures. In many areas of society – farming, for example, or privately-owned business – children are a parent's best hope of on-going prosperity, of land tenure or of commercial continuity.

More powerful still are the genetic pressures. These are expressed in sexuality, in the urges of coitus, in the love of family, in the deep affection for our own kind that is so intimate a part of our behaviour. The very foundations of our nature, these pressures lie deep in the history of humanity's evolution. Once they ensured the survival of the species in a hostile world. Only two hundred years ago around three-quarters of all children born in Britain were dead by the age of five – so it's hardly surprising, with women producing an average of eight children at most during their relatively short reproductive lives, that the urge to breed has had to be so all-consuming. Today, of course, on a world scale this urge has got us into serious trouble, but it's still with us, the result of an evolutionary time-lag, and on an individual level we have a responsibility to understand and accept it.

Darwin knew these drives well enough, and the importance of maximising reproduction for species to survive. His modern disciples elaborate his ideas, endlessly fascinated by the patterns of sexual selection.

'Sexual behaviour, an essential part of the total behavioural repertoire of every higher organism . . .' wrote two of them, F. von Schilcher and N. Tennant. 'Evolutionary genetics has always recognised the "evolutionary sense" of parents' caring for offspring, even at cost to themselves, as the genes' way of ensuring further propagation.'

One of their fellow behaviourists, Desmond Morris, even seeks to explain biologically the mystery of falling in love:

'For a virile primate to go off on a feeding trip and leave his female unprotected from the advances of other males that might happen by was unheard-of . . . The answer was the development of a pair-bond . . . to fall in love and remain faithful to one another . . .' For the parenthood of a child has clearly been deeply significant both on a personal and on a tribal level since the beginning of social organisation, and only by sexual faithfulness could it be assured.

Again, beyond pair-bonding or 'falling in love', there is the most powerful force of all: love itself, enduring and complex. Love for a wife, a husband, a child. How desperately an infertile woman may long to feel and express love in this most natural and fundamental way! It is the stuff of poetry, of music and drama, of transcendence. It's also a matter of the vast stores of biological energy locked in the menstrual cycle, in men's and women's acute awareness of their reproductive apparatus, in the strength of sexual attraction and the delirium of the orgasm. A formidable combination of forces indeed. Who can be surprised at their power, or censure the need to satisfy their urgings?

Some people respond to these inner pressures strongly, others hardly at all. Neither group should be judged. Sometimes a man or a woman seems to long for fertility because they love their child even before it is conceived. Thus, realisation of their infertility can cause grief, often needing a long period of recovery. On other occasions a mother's love flowers so vividly that one accidentally given another's baby in hospital may be fiercely unwilling to accept the child that is biologically hers, even when the error is quickly discovered. Passions can run very high, and society is rightly sympathetic. In August, 1986, when confusion arose over two little boys born within ten minutes of each other in an Irish hospital, the *Daily Mail* didn't exaggerate when it told its readers: 'Did they take the wrong babies home from the maternity hospital? . . . Two distraught mothers were waiting last night for the answer to a nightmare question.'

We may laugh. We may find it inconvenient, impossible to square with the tidy solutions we'd like to impose. But the fact undeniably remains that for very many men and women the deep genetic need exists for a child that is perceived to be in some immediate physical sense their own, *of their own blood*. For such people, should they be infertile, adoption is no solution. Their need is for a child related to them in its genes — and therefore to a degree in its physical characteristics, or its talents, or even its sense of humour — so that it can be understood and loved and guided with a special closeness as it grows to adulthood. Perhaps this is the need Plato was thinking of two thousand years ago, when he wrote, 'There is a sense in which nature has not only endowed the human race with a degree of immortality, but has also implanted in us all a longing to achieve it, which we express in every way we can.'

This is one answer, then, to those people who suggest banning the abortion of unwanted babies in order to make them available for adoption. But the idea, anyway, is quite monstrous. The proposal is to deny medical treatment to one set of people simply in order to solve another group's problem. The proposal is to compel unwilling women to continue their pregnancies, with all the discomfort and danger this involves, and then to go through the considerable trauma of labour and delivery, simply in order to give the baby away immediately to someone else. Possibly such anti-abortionists have thoughts of punishment for what they see as sin when they make this proposal. Certainly they threaten individual human dignity and freedom far more than the practice of in-vitro fertilisation ever can.

The mention of sin brings us to the involvement of the churches. We may live in an avowedly secular age, but the influence of the churches on public opinion, and often on legislation, is still very pervasive. Although unfashionable, the Biblical injunction to 'be fruitful and multiply' has been drummed into congregation upon congregation, in ceremonies of marriage, christening, and in regular weekly services, so that the message lies deep in every Christian's conscience and must bear heavily upon the infertile.

Up to now on the particular issue of IVF, the Church of England has been on the side of thoughtful argument, uncertain rather than dogmatic. Its Board of Social Responsibility has formed a specially appointed working party which has issued an interim report: it fears that scientists may lose a sense of the boundaries of natural law and thus obscure God's purpose, but it accepts that change is inevitable. 'The creative process continues and involves ever-widening horizons of human knowledge and capability. We are in the midst of a journey whose beginnings lay in creation and whose end is to be realised in the hope given to us in Jesus Christ.'

The report accepts that love can be expressed through contraception, and that procreation and sexual intercourse can be separated without the loss of any fundamental truth. It also accepts 'assisted fertilisation' if it holds together the relationship of marriage. 'One may say that the procreation of children is not just an optional matter for Christians. It is a proper goal of marriage, intended by the ordinance of the Creator himself . . .'

Other churches are less sympathetic. An American Baptist, Paul Ramsay, has stood out strongly against IVF for many years. For one thing, he says, the necessary sperm has to be obtained by means of masturbation which is immoral, and for another, scientists who conceive embryos outside the human body are playing God: 'Only an unexamined preference for *human design* over nature can support any other conclusion,' he wrote in the *Journal of the American Medical Association.*

The Roman Catholic Church is more extreme in its condemnation. Children must be conceived in wedlock through sexual intercourse: this is the only way, so artificial insemination and test-tube babies will never do. The Congregation for the Doctrine of the Faith of the Vatican wrote in 1987 that, 'Conception in vitro is the result of a technical action.' It then went on in italics, 'Such fertilisation is neither in fact achieved nor positively willed as the expression and fruit of a specific act of the conjugal union . . . Such fertilisation is in itself illicit and in opposition to the dignity of procreation and of the conjugal union . . .'

Another report by Roman Catholic bishops claims: 'To have or procreate a child by IVF is a choice in which the child does not have the status which a child of sexual union has . . . Unlike other children, IVF children cannot say, "I have my origin in a single act, an act of love or friendship or mutual involvement and commitment, an act equally of each of my parents and of themselves alone; an act by which they submitted themselves to each other and to the source of human life."'

I find these remarks singularly misguided. Can parental intention really alter the 'status' — whatever that may mean — of children? Aren't the bishops really suffering the little children to come to them only in order that they may be told how unequal they are, how much better or how much worse?

Perhaps this is a minority view within the Roman Catholic Church. I hope it is. But the pernicious attitudes it exemplifies rub off on society at large, and I and many other scientists working in my field have been at the receiving end of similar bigotries for a long time. The accusations against us are various. Many centre on the evils of self-indulgence. We are told we do not cure infertility, we simply pander to the vanity or possessiveness of our patients. In the strictest sense, we do not 'cure' infertility — and neither do spectacles, insulin, false teeth or aspirin 'cure' the conditions they treat. Like them, in-vitro fertilisation relieves unpleasant and sometimes tragic symptoms. I see nothing unworthy or self-indulgent in that, either for doctor or patient.

Sometimes, on the other hand, we are told that we're pushing on with an advance that will harm the stable structures of society, for IVF will enable single women, or even homosexuals, to have children. This is nonsense. The huge majority of single women, and of homosexuals of either sex, can have children quite well without our help. They're perfectly fertile. They have no need of IVF: the issue for them is whether to accept artificial insemination or a sex act gone through for procreation's sake, against their erotic inclinations — the ethics of which, being mercifully outside the law, they decide for themselves.

Fortunately, for married couples at any rate, wisdom concerning the acceptance of IVF has generally prevailed in successive commissions, committees and governments across the world. The Warnock Committee, appointed in Britain to assess the ethics of the matter, arrived at the following conclusion in 1984: 'Medicine is no longer exclusively concerned with the preservation of life, but also with remedying the malfunctions of the human body. On this analysis, an inability to have children is a malfunction and should be considered in exactly the same way as any other . . . Infertility is not something mysterious, nor a cause for shame, nor necessarily something that has to be endured without attempted cure . . . The psychological distress that may be caused by infertility in those who want children may precipitate a mental disorder warranting treatment . . .'

So, why do I bother with infertility? I have 'bothered with infertility' for most of my working life, because I see in it a cause of great and lasting human sadness. It demands treatment. People have a right, I believe, to benefit from research whenever possible, and there is no reason to think that ethical advice from outsiders about their actions is sounder than their own judgment. They must receive treatment if they ask for it because great dangers lurk in the restriction or witholding of any medical procedure on grounds of religion, or expense, or anything else. If the access of my patients to a remedy is impaired, so might the access of others be, with different illnesses.

The treatment involved in IVF is not something that couples undertake lightly. Enormous determination and dedication are required, great hope and perseverance, and the courage to accept repeated disappointments. But I have seen patients' joy, their radiant faces when the news I give them is good, and I know that not one of them would say the effort hadn't been worth it. And if they can say that, then so can I.

Finally, on this subject I remember the words of Barbara Amiel, who wrote in *The Times* for 3 April 1987, 'A nice woman in a starched uniform told me . . . that I was unable to have a child . . . As she spoke, all I could see was a large black crow sitting on her shoulder. The crow just sat there, its beak hard, yellow, ready to gnaw out my insides . . .'

So that is why I bother with infertility. And that, or some faintly heard, faintly understood echo of it, is why society at large has accepted the need for in-vitro fertilisation as a suitable, if controversial treatment. The alternative is a large black crow, its beak hard and yellow, sitting on a childless woman's shoulder.

Now the argument has moved on from the rights and

wrongs of IVF, and different battle lines are being drawn all over the world: the rights and wrongs of embryo research instead, of frozen embryos, of gamete and embryo donation, of surrogate motherhood. Positions become entrenched as debate gives way to abuse and the opposing war-cries are vainly repeated. But society will eventually have to choose between the various camps, and what society still needs, most of all, is information.

A few facts, therefore, before I get on to questions of morals or ethics or government legislation. What, for example, actually goes on in an IVF clinic?

# 3
# Life in a Busy IVF Clinic

These days there must be literally hundreds of test-tube baby clinics, located in countries all round the world. Some exist as specialist departments, often tiny, set up in general hospitals or private nursing homes, while others — like ours at Bourn Hall — are large and completely self-sufficient. The standard of accommodation varies similarly, from the spartan to the frankly luxurious. Nevertheless, if they are to function properly they will all be staffed by the same basic personnel of highly skilled nurses, doctors and scientists, they will have access to the same range of wards, laboratories and theatres, and they will offer the same procedures.

The patients' first contact used to be with the clinic's consulting gynaecologist, although more often today with a new-styled Nurse Coordinator, who stays close to the couple throughout their treatment, counselling, advising and treating. Usually both husband and wife attend an initial visit. The specialist sizes them up as they enter his consulting room. He has their records on his desk in front of him, but he also searches for some evidence with his own eyes and ears as in the following imaginary scene.

'Good morning, Mrs Dawson . . . Mr Dawson. Sit down, please.' This is a taxing, anxious interview for the Dawsons and the consultant makes a point of being relaxed and friendly. 'Let's see if we can help in some way with your problem. And the first thing I need to know is, how long has this infertility been bothering you?'

This is an important question. The couple will have been referred to the clinic by their own doctor, but even so some consultants refuse to treat patients unless they have been trying for a child for at least two years. Unless their infertility is very long and firmly established it is well known that couples may conceive perfectly naturally, perhaps even within a few days of their first consultation, without receiving any treatment at all. Infertility is imperfectly understood – sometimes it seems to be cured simply by going through a sympathetic consultant's door!

'We've been trying for over five years,' comes Mrs Dawson's sad reply. 'We've been under the care of Doctor Williams – he's sent us to see you.'

Five years . . . the specialist recognises her desperation, all the hopelessness and isolation of her and her husband's situation, the endless consultations, probably with a succession of doctors, and the unvarying failures.

'That's a long time, Mrs Dawson. I can see now why you're here – obviously you've tried all the more usual methods, so maybe in-vitro fertilisation will be just the thing . . .' He pauses as his patients settle down, smile at each other nervously. 'Now then – how old are you, Mrs Dawson?'

This is another important question. Many couples fail to turn to IVF until the woman is approaching forty, by which time – even in the most fertile of women – her fertility will be declining. Older women also have a greater chance of losing their pregnancy than younger women, whether it's established normally or by IVF. But Mrs Dawson turns out to be thirty-two, so the consultant is well pleased.

He needs a lot more information. He knows Mrs Dawson's medical records, but confirms with her much of what he finds there. Does she ovulate? Are her periods regular? Has she ever been pregnant before, in an earlier marriage perhaps? Has she had any major operations? Are there organs in her abdomen that adhere, to complicate the collection of her eggs? Is her blood rhesus negative? Is she allergic to any particular drugs or hormones? Has she suffered from any serious diseases?

When all these questions have been answered satisfactorily, the consultant turns to Mr Dawson. Has he had difficulty with reproduction before, with a previous wife, say? Has he had a fertility check-up recently? If so, does he produce few spermatozoa, or spermatozoa that are abnormally formed? If Mr and Mrs Dawson have been consulting doctors about their fertility for some time, by now Mr Dawson will have got used to such questions and will not consider them insulting as many men do, or aspersions on his virility. In fact his answers are satisfactory too, and the sperm count given in his records is adequate, so the Dawsons look like excellent prospects for successful IVF.

Before the specialist will commit himself a few further routine tests are necessary. All couples are tested for AIDS, for example, since they could not be treated if either were positive – AIDS can damage a fetus in its mother's womb, condemning it to a brief, wretched existence. Their general health is checked, too.

A few days later, after the results of all the tests are through, Mr and Mrs Dawson return to the clinic.

'So far so good,' the consultant tells them. 'Now we must decide on the exact nature of your treatment. Nowadays there are several possibilities – it could be in-vitro fertilisation . . . or GIFT . . . or maybe DIPI. But before I blind you with too much science, let's talk about the causes of your own particular infertility.'

Mrs Dawson's Fallopian tubes might be blocked, or her husband might have a low sperm count. She might have immunity against his spermatozoa, or internal adhesions, or she might suffer from endometriosis – the displacement of uterine cells which can be suppressed by steroids. Blocked Fallopian tubes are one of the most usual causes of infertility, however – they prevent an egg or embryo from passing into its mother's womb from her ovary, and they can be damaged by infection, by inflammation, or even by surgery dating back many years. Clearly such infertility can afflict even the most exemplary of women, yet there are moralists who claim it must be the result of some misdemeanour such as teenage promiscuity or illegal abortion, and therefore is a just retribution and should not be cured.

Ignoring such vengeful nonsense, if his patient's tubes *are* blocked, the specialist must consider if he can repair them, opening their delicate channels to embryonic life again. If repair is impossible, then in-vitro fertilisation is necessary. And this turns out to be the situation in Mrs Dawson's case.

'All our examinations show that your tubes are hopelessly blocked,' he tells her, 'so I'm recommending in-vitro fertilisation. For this we'll need several of your eggs, of course − and to be sure of these we'll give you one or other of the well-tried fertility drugs, like clomiphene or HMG. This will stimulate a number of follicles to grow, providing us with plenty of eggs. We'll withdraw the eggs by means of ultrasound when the time comes. It doesn't hurt at all, and we don't even have to keep you here in the clinic overnight . . .'

The consultant reaches for his pad. 'Here's your prescription. Off you go now − and don't worry. Just start the medicine the day after your menstrual period begins. And we'll book you in here for an ultrasound a week or so after that. So keep in touch. And good luck!'

Other possibilities exist. The consultant might decide to take more time, to use new drugs that quieten down the reproductive cycle initially so that the older drugs may then be given more effectively. To avoid fertilisation failures in his culture dishes he needs a minimum of seven or eight eggs, and these modern treatments stimulate some patients' egg production very successfully − even as many as fifty-five eggs have been obtained occasionally.

Since each fertilised egg only has a 10−15 per cent chance of implanting in its mother, most clinics now ideally replace three or four, thus raising the chances of a pregnancy. With two eggs replaced, 25 per cent of women become pregnant, and 20 per cent of these have twins. With three fertilised eggs, up to 30% of women become pregnant. We at Bourn Hall have sometimes tried replacing four, hoping to improve still further the chances of pregnancy — but we're careful to make it clear to patients that their chances of triplets are higher in such circumstances, and even, very rarely, quadruplets.

The chances of pregnancy seem lower in certain clinics, so some specialists replace five or six, even as many as twelve, in a desperate attempt to achieve a pregnancy. The risk, of course, is that excessively multiple pregnancies may result — quintuplet fetuses, even more, have arisen already, so such gynaecologists may well plan in advance to destroy all but two or three — and I have to say that the ethics of choosing between unwanted fetuses and 'culling' three or four seem to me extremely doubtful. I myself would never replace so many.

In any case, Mr and Mrs Dawson depart quite cheerfully, anticipating no such difficulties and cheered by their prospects.

The consultant's next patients are Mr and Mrs Roberts. All this couple's tests have been completed and he knows that, as well as the wife, the husband too has a problem. They enter the room uncertainly, suspecting that they have a difficult decision ahead.

Referring to his notes, the consultant confirms their worst fears. 'I'm afraid, Mr Roberts, that besides your wife's damaged tubes, it may well be that you yourself have too few spermatozoa to achieve fertilisation . . . Last time you were here we discussed what might be done if that were the case. I mentioned the possibility of using spermatozoa from a donor for an in-vitro fertilisation. You said you'd think it over . . .'

Mrs Roberts reaches for her husband's hand. Obviously they have discussed the question long and often. But it is still no easy matter.

'We've almost made up our minds,' Mr Roberts answers.

'But we'd like more advice. You said you could choose a donor with my height and more or less my looks – but we'd still much rather try for our own child. Can't we do both? Wouldn't this give us the best chance of our own baby? Or maybe have a try with just my spermatozoa first? Tell us what you think.'

The consultant hesitates, weighing the odds. He knows that the embryologist in his laboratory will conserve and treasure the few spermatozoa that Mr Roberts produces, and will introduce them as favourably as possible to his wife's eggs in their dish of culture medium. But supposing none becomes fertilised, what then? The entire egg-gathering procedure will have been wasted and Mrs Roberts' morale, already poor, will drop to a new low. She'll have to go home, disappointed yet again, and more weeks will have to pass.

Another possibility, suggested by Mr Roberts, is that half of her eggs be cultured with his spermatozoa, and the other half with the donor's. Certainly this prolongs Mr Roberts' hopes. But if it doesn't succeed it also increases his sense of failure. Alternatively, Mr Roberts' spermatozoa could be added to her eggs first, and the donor's a few hours later. All her eggs might then be fertilised by her husband, but they might all be fertilised by the donor, and nobody would be able to tell for certain which had happened. Some couples might prefer this course, but not, the consultant believes, Mr and Mrs Roberts.

'Let's wait to find out how many eggs you have, Mrs Roberts,' he says. 'If there are enough we'll inseminate half with your husband's spermatozoa and half with the donor's. That seems to me best. But it's up to you, of course – do you agree?'

They talk some more, but the decision has been made really and – like Mrs Dawson – Mrs Roberts eventually goes away with her prescription for fertility drugs.

Following their menstrual periods both women attend the clinic regularly, so that their responses can be monitored by ultrasound. This is simple and quite painless: they simply lie very still as a scanner is passed over their abdomens, sending pictures of their developing follicles onto a screen. These are seen to be growing steadily larger. And since each follicle releases hormones into the blood, their levels rise steadily too, and are monitored. With such powerful diagnostic tools few mistakes are made, and the exact number of growing follicles in each woman is soon identified.

Mrs Dawson receives good news.

'A very nice response,' the ultrasonographer tells her, eight days after she has begun taking the medicine. 'Seven follicles — maybe even eight. Look — you can see them for yourself. And your hormone levels are doing fine, too.'

Mrs Roberts isn't quite so lucky. She has only four follicles, but at least each is growing well, and their hormones are showing up in her blood. Even so, being already aware of her husband's low sperm count, she understandably begins to worry.

At this stage, unless their hormone levels are watched very carefully, either woman might just possibly react adversely to her treatment by ovulating. In that case all her eggs would be lost, shed uselessly into her abdomen. So their hormonal balance is checked daily, by collecting samples of urine as often as eight times each day. For Mrs Dawson and Mrs Roberts, fortunately, there are no undesirable developments. On the tenth day of testing everything is seen to be stable and satisfactory. A hormone specialist tells the two women that the clinic is ready to induce their ovulation. They will be given the drug HCG that evening, and their ripe eggs will be collected thirty-six hours later. Semen will be required from their husbands three hours before that.

This is how the stage is set, by careful observation and the harnessing of natural processes, for the next stage in their treatment, the in-vitro fertilisation itself. But here too the times are changing, and new synthetic hormones,

ultrasound, and 'programming' cycles are simplifying matters. Waiting for nature to take its course is no longer
necessary: the day and even the virtual hour of egg
collection can be arranged in advance. 'Never on a Sunday!'
wrote the French Doctor Zorn, describing one such
programme in the *Lancet*.

Interestingly, in spite of all these changes, over the last
thirty years one factor has remained constant: the drug I
gave to those mice in Edinburgh to induce their ovulation
was the same as is used today: HCG. It causes eggs to ripen
in an entirely predictable way – in a mouse after eleven
hours, in a woman after thirty-seven. Once each egg has
grown sufficiently on its follicle, therefore, the cycle is
controllable and complete. And this is the pattern that
patients come to know: first a fertility drug such as
clomiphene on the first day of their menstrual period, then
HMG to make their follicles grow, with meticulous
observations as their follicles and eggs develop, then HCG
when the moment is right.

Many clinics offer treatment on an out-patient basis,
which may be more convenient for working couples, and
certainly helps to keep costs down. But the constant
travelling can be stressful, and critical decisions have to be
taken at very short notice in the final days before HCG is
administered – decisions that may require a very sensitive
hormone check or the taking of another ultrasound scan –
so that there are clinics (like ours at Bourn Hall) that
strongly recommend in-patient status, at least in the final
stages.

At last, for Mrs Dawson, the moment is right and HCG
has done its work. 'It's time to collect your eggs now,' the
surgeon tells her. 'We'll be using ultrasound, so you won't
need a general anaesthetic. You can easily have one,
though, if you'd prefer it.'

In the old days, collecting the eggs by means of
laparoscopy usually required general anaesthesia. Using
ultrasound, however, surgeons can guide a fine needle

across the vaginal wall into each follicle in turn, gently withdrawing its contents into a collecting dish, and all with the use of only a minor local anaesthetic in many patients. This is now a very popular procedure, for a woman's eggs can be collected in twenty minutes, and she is back to normal a few hours later, and with very little discomfort. Understandably, however, some women don't like the idea of this, and prefer to be unconscious as their follicles are aspirated.

Mrs Dawson chooses local anaesthesia, and is keenly interested as the surgeon empties her follicles one by one. 'How many eggs do I have?' she asks the embryologist anxiously, as her ultrasound is finished.

The embryologist studies each sample under his microscope. The eggs in them are excellent, every one surrounded by nurse cells and a small blob of protective jelly. 'There are ten eggs, all healthy,' he tells her. 'They're all ripe and ready for fertilisation.'

He takes the eggs and places them in dishes in the incubator. 'There should be no difficulty with fertilisation. Your husband's spermatozoa are fine and active — they'll quickly penetrate your eggs.'

He will add spermatozoa to the eggs soon afterwards, and fertilisation will take place over the next twenty-four hours. A day or two after that the eggs will develop into embryos, to be replaced in their mother via a very fine tube which is passed through her vagina, her cervix, and into her womb. For most women the procedure takes around thirty seconds, without any anaesthesia, and some women remain unaware that anything has been done to them.

Mrs Roberts is next. For her, too, the HCG has done its work and each of her four follicles yields a healthy ripening egg. But she has to be told that there are still problems, since her husband's spermatozoa are as sparse (in reproductive terms) as the consultant had feared.

But Mr and Mrs Roberts have talked it over and made up their minds. 'If my four eggs are healthy,' Mrs Roberts says to the embryologist, 'then add my husband's sperm to two of them, and the donor's to the other two. I know that cuts down on the chances, but we do so much want to have a baby together if we can.' Their decision also avoided any problems arising by adding his sperm first to all the eggs, and the donor sperm a few hours later. The identity of the child would be uncertain, which might be an illegal act in some countries, and some doctors feel that mixed inseminations like this mean that the patients have not really accepted the implications of donor insemination.

The embryologist looks through his microscope at the sperm in their fluid. There are few of them and they are not particularly active. He does what Mrs Roberts has asked him to, but he doubts if they will fertilise. The donor's sperm, on the other hand, are excellent.

Another patient is brought in. She is having DIPI. Her tubes are not blocked, and her treatment is almost over. She has four follicles, also, and the embryologist makes up a suspension of around five million of her husband's spermatozoa. Such numbers may sound huge, but nature is prodigal and the wastage built into all its reproductive processes is enormous. The surgeon takes the mixture of eggs and sperm and injects it into the patient's abdomen. The procedure is still experimental, but very often a woman's tubes will draw in her ovulatory eggs and the sperm through their own powerful currents of fluid and a pregnancy will result.

Yet another patient arrives. Her tubes are also open, and she is having GIFT. She has supplied the embryologist with twelve eggs. He selects four of the better eggs, mixes them with a half-million or so of her husband's sperm, and the surgeon places them delicately in her oviduct, using a laparoscope. The other eight eggs are inseminated in-vitro – the embryologist intends to freeze any embryos that result, in case they're needed later.

It has been a typical morning. The last two patients were lucky, having tubes healthy enough to sustain fertilisation and carry embryos to the womb. As for Mrs Dawson and Mrs Roberts, their eggs are inseminated and in the incubator now, where they will stay overnight. If all goes well active spermatozoa will be penetrating between the nurse cells in an hour or two, separating them from the eggs. The sperm will reach the egg membrane and a few will attach to it, as a temporary resting place. After a further hour or so one or two sperm may become violently active, thrusting in, creating a tiny slit in the membrane. Within a few minutes one or both will touch the egg itself, slowing their activity as they fuse gently with it. The gametes have come together and the first stages of fertilisation are complete.

During the night two nuclei — called pronuclei — appear in healthily fertilised eggs. One comes from the spermatozöon and the other from the mother's chromosomes, an equal contribution from each parent, and a clear sign that embryonic life has begun.

It still has a long way to go. Implantation remains a very uncertain process. Nobody yet knows why, but an apparently viable embryo is three times less likely to develop successfully after IVF than in a couple conceiving naturally. In 1985 the Voluntary Licensing Authority in Britain had licensed twenty-five IVF clinics, and overall averages of successful pregnancies resulting from a single treatment episode stood at around 8.9 per cent. This is of course only an average; some clinics were — and still are — achieving 25 per cent success rates, while those of others are substantially lower. Needless to say, the low rate of pregnancy attracts critical press comment, especially in North America. But in any case, the average couple makes three attempts at IVF and, if they have been properly counselled and selected in the first place, many are eventually successful.

Thus, although the first signs of embryonic life are clearly only the beginnings of a long and perilous journey, it is a journey well worth attempting.

The following morning the embryologist examines all

the eggs he has left in the incubator. Of Mrs Dawson's ten eggs, nine have two superb pronuclei, each normally fertilised. The tenth, however, has three pronuclei. It has been fertilised by two spermatozoa and will grow abnormally, with too many chromosomes. It will not survive, just as it would not have survived in the natural state, if it had arisen through normal intercourse. Still, Mrs Dawson has nine fertile, healthy eggs, so she need not worry.

The embryologist turns to Mrs Roberts's eggs. As he feared, her husband's spermatozoa have failed: those two of her eggs have no pronuclei at all. Anxiously he examines the other two: both are fertilised; each has two pronuclei. He relaxes: the donor's spermatozoa have succeeded. The pronucleate eggs could be replaced in the mother's womb straight away, and some clinics actually do this, but most wait one more day, to make sure the embryos are growing well.

Thirdly, the eight eggs of the patient receiving GIFT. These are fertilised too, and in a few days will be ready for freezing. So, although Mrs Roberts will be disappointed, there's a measure of good news for all three women.

Each pronucleate egg has the possibility – if all goes well – of becoming a child. The embryologist transfers the eggs to fresh droplets of culture medium, and then returns them to the incubator. And by the next day the embryos should be well formed. The two pronuclei have moved together and their chromosomes have intermingled. The eggs have then divided into two equal parts, and become 2-cell embryos. Some may have gone further, and divided into four cells.

The embryologist examines Mrs Dawson's nine embryos. There they are, exactly on time, 2-cell embryos growing excellently . . . or does one look sick? One of its cells seems too big – is it growing wrongly? He examines the other eight again and chooses four which are already 4-cell, to be replaced in her womb later that day.

Mrs Roberts's two embryos are both growing well, and

will be ready for replacement too. And the eight embryos of the GIFT case are flourishing also.

He rings the nurse. 'Tell Mrs Dawson and Mrs Roberts we'll be ready to replace their embryos this evening. They're looking very good indeed.'

This is the news that all patients long for, and at least four-fifths of them receive it in a good clinic. I only wish their chances of a successful pregnancy after replacement were equally good. But research is continuous, and rates are improving all the time.

That evening the embryologist is back on duty. 'Eight lovely embryos, Mrs Dawson,' he tells her as she waits for her replacement. 'The ninth didn't grow very well, I'm afraid, and the tenth was fertilized by two spermatozoa and couldn't have survived. I suggest we replace four, and freeze the other four in case you should need them later.'

She agrees. Then she asks what for her is the most important question of all: 'What are my chances of pregnancy, then?'

He pauses, determined to be truthful. 'With four embryos you have as much as a 35 per cent chance of pregnancy, Mrs Dawson. Each embryo is fine, and you yourself are young and in excellent health. Also, since you have no record of miscarriages or abortions in the past, if you should become pregnant you stand a very good chance indeed of sustaining the pregnancy.'

He pats her hand, then returns to his laboratory where he loads the four embryos he has chosen into a delicate, specially supple catheter. This he carries to the surgeon, who threads it gently through Mrs Dawson's cervical canal and into her womb. Equally gently the embryologist depresses the syringe, expressing her embryos in a tiny droplet of fluid into her womb, back into their mother.

In his terms she's been a very good patient. Other women may supply more eggs, but many of these fragment, or grow unevenly, or simply fail to grow at all. He doesn't really understand what makes this happen. Obviously some malformed embryos must carry the wrong chromosomes, like the egg fertilised by two spermatozoa. Others may have been fertilised too late, or may carry a disabling gene. But there's a lot he still doesn't know.

Now Mrs Roberts is waiting, disappointed by the failure of her husband's spermatozoa but delighted all the same with her two healthy embryos. Her replacement goes smoothly too.

That leaves the eggs awaiting freezing to be dealt with, and Mrs Dawson's two unsuccessful embryos. These will have to be thrown away or used for research. Two small tragedies, he tells himself. Tragedies indeed, but un-avoidable, and very small in the grand scale of nature's design. Their loss is balanced by the hopes of life that their healthier companions have brought.

Mrs Dawson and Mrs Roberts rest for a few hours after their replacements. They have been in or at the clinic now probably for three or four days and their treatment is almost over. There are no tests to monitor an embryo's progress immediately after it has been replaced in its mother. For all the experts know, it may have died the moment it entered its mother's womb. Or it may have been expelled from her by a simple involuntary muscular spasm — especially if her hormonal balance turns out to have been not quite right for the support of a pregnancy. Everybody simply has to wait patiently for a sign in the mother that one or more of her embryos has implanted and is searching her tissues for nourishment and oxygen.

'Goodbye and good luck,' the nurse at the desk says as the two women depart, 'and don't forget — we'll want you back for a drop of blood in fifteen days, to find out if you are pregnant.' In fact, the first reliable sign of pregnancy comes about ten days after fertilisation. Implanted embryos now release a hormone into their mother's blood as a clear sign of their vitality. Thus a blood test now or a day or so later will confirm the pregnancy beyond all doubt.

Mrs Dawson's blood sample arrives on day 15. It proves

to be negative – she isn't pregnant, and her treatment has failed. At a subsequent appointment the consultant tells her and her husband, 'I really am so very sorry your embryos didn't implant. But it's one of those things – we don't yet understand properly why some women become pregnant and others don't. Of course, we can always try again if you like. There's nothing to stop you.'

For a moment the Dawsons are distressed, their confidence gone, their faith in science shattered. Then Mrs Dawson remembers her frozen embryos.

'But, Doctor – what about those four embryos of mine you froze? Can't I have them replaced during my next cycle?' she asks, hoping to avoid the delay and bother of further treatments with fertility drugs and ultrasound. 'I want to try again with them as soon as possible, please.'

'I don't see why not,' the consultant replies. 'Three-quarters of all good embryos survive thawing well, so your chances will be pretty high.'

Their hopes rise again at this second chance of a pregnancy, and with so little hassle. A single short visit, that's all that will be needed, during which the thawed-out embryos will be replaced in Mrs Dawson's womb.

They prepare to leave. On their way out they meet Mrs Roberts, who is ecstatic. One of her two embryos has implanted, she is pregnant, and all her apprehensions have flown.

There are other patients out in the waiting room, heavily pregnant women who have been treated months before and who are back at the clinic for an ante-natal check-up. But there may also be patients even more disappointed than the Dawsons, women who perhaps have successfully conceived only to miscarry at six weeks, or even at three months, just when everything seemed to be going well. For reasons we don't yet understand one-fifth of all test-tube pregnancies end this way.

No chapter on IVF clinics would be complete without a mention of cost. At the time of writing there are a few excellent, and free, NHS clinics. Most of these will only accept patients from within their own regions, and even then severe funding restrictions are producing waiting lists of two years and more – and some of the university-funded health service clinics even make a small charge also, possibly in the region of £250. In many countries of Europe and in Australia, state insurance schemes bear most of the costs. In the private sector all over the world, charges for such sophisticated treatment are inevitably high: with such close in-patient care as in Bourn Hall, somewhere between £1500 and £2000 at one time. Costs are less now with more simplified treatments. These are realistic estimates for each full treatment cycle, including the costs of freezing embryos and at such figures there are probably no great fortunes being made.

This, then, is day-to-day life in an IVF clinic. Couples trying for a pregnancy have to be very patient and determined. But the treatments offer an excellent chance of success, and are now generally accepted by society as both moral and beneficial. It is on the subject of future lines of research, principally, and in matters such as surrogate pregnancies, that the moral issues become more clouded. Before I get to these, there are many more facts, especially about embryonic growth, to be properly discussed and understood.

For example, ethicists, legislators and churchmen use the phrase *the human embryo* a very great deal these days. Yet it is by no means certain just what they mean by it.

# 4
# The Human Embryo
# 1. A definition

What is an embryo, when does it arise, and when does it turn into a fetus? Answers to these questions ought to be simple. In fact they are extraordinarily complex. Even so, they must be tackled before any later questions can be faced.

The confusions begin where they might least be expected, with the professionals, the doctors and the scientists. Doctors tend to think of an embryo as beginning at fertilisation and not becoming a fetus until most organs are formed, by which time it is clearly human in shape and characteristics. Many scientists, on the other hand, place the change to fetus much earlier, when the organism is still minute and unformed, without even a front or a rear, a right or a left side. Much unnecessary public revulsion may be attributed to this confusion, as a doctor's substantial two-month-old embryo is mistakenly pictured when research is reported on what is in fact a scientist's microscopic two-week-old embryo, and images arise of tiny human beings reacting in pain as they are exposed to experimental drugs or noxious agents.

This simply does not happen. Embryo research of the kind I will describe is carried out on only the earliest of living embryos. In the first few days of its development a

cleaving embryo reaches sixteen cells, looks like a microscopic raspberry, and is properly called a morula. Four days
later, still scarcely larger than the unfertilised egg, its cells
have begun to specialise and it is called a blastocyst. Two
weeks after this it is still almost invisible to the naked eye,
and it will not be even remotely recognisable as human for a
further three weeks – long before which time virtually all
conceivably useful research will have been completed.

Even so there are those who claim that such early
research is unjustified, that embryos in every one of those
stages should be given the same rights and privileges as an
adult human.

I don't want to get caught up in detailed ethical issues in
this chapter. But it must be said that society at large does
not seem to support this absolutist position: society readily
demotes embryonic life every time it sanctions intra-uterine
or morning-after contraceptives which expel from their
mothers embryos aged five days or more, or accepts
interceptives and contragestives which remove life support
from embryos of fourteen days and older. Its tolerance of
abortion, too, suggests a willingness to regard the unborn
in some important senses as less than human.

The battle over embryos' rights isn't entirely lost,
however. Under British law an embryo can inherit its
father's estate if he dies while it's in its mother's womb, and
if it goes on to be born alive. It can also claim damages for
injury inflicted while in the womb, provided that it lives for
forty-eight hours after its birth. Not that it can do either, of
course, if it has been scraped off the womb by an intra-
uterine device, or discarded by a post-coital pill, which
might be thought the ultimate of injuries.

In short, society is confused. But so is the situation.

The absolutists do their best. The Roman Catholic
Church and such watchdog organisations associated with
the anti-abortion lobby as LIFE try to clarify matters by
asserting that sperm and eggs, as long as they are kept
apart, are of no moral significance, but that once they come

together the outcome is sacrosanct. Egg plus sperm equals human life. No matter what benefits might result, research on human embryos is therefore immoral, since each time it occurs a human being is tampered with or killed. This argument seems simple. It is easily understood, and it gains force and credibility by determined repetition. But its simplicity is in fact a fake.

The absolutist's argument centres on the moment of fertilisation. Before fertilisation, an egg and a sperm: after fertilisation, human life. All human rights therefore mature at that moment. This is either a scientific argument or it is nothing. No biblical guidance sustains the notion of sudden human existence, let alone sudden human rights, as an egg is fertilised. Indeed, theologians admit to difficulty in deciding exactly when the human soul enters the embryo, separating human from non-human life.

So this is a scientific argument, and scientific arguments depend upon meticulous observation, upon fact rather than faith. Ethics similarly depend upon fact, upon accurate information and free access to such information. If one fact undermines an ethical stance, the whole edifice crumbles.

Fertilisation, then — what is it? A remarkable process certainly, exciting and inspiring, but hardly magical. Evolution discovered its advantages millennia ago: it promotes viability, shuffling the available genes into endless new combinations. Whether it occurs in man, fish or frog, these genes combine as a spermatozoön fuses with an egg, and meticulous observation tells us that this fusing takes place in distinct stages.

Egg plus sperm . . . First of all, a spermatozoön binds on to the lifeless outer membrane of the egg. Is this the decisive moment which confers full human status? No: the egg is still inert and if nothing else happens it will never become an embryo.

Minutes later, perhaps a quarter of an hour, the sperm penetrates the membrane and touches the egg itself. Is this the moment? No: between them the egg and the sperm now have far too many chromosomes, and unless they expel one-third of them (which they will do in an hour or two) normal development will not continue. Also, at this stage a second spermatozoön can still enter the egg, causing uncertainty as to whether life began with the first or the second.

Egg plus sperm . . . Undeniably fertilisation is under way now, but human life still will not be the outcome until other stages have been passed. Two or three hours later the surplus chromosomes have been expelled and no more spermatozoa can enter the egg. Is this the moment? No: the mother's and father's chromosomes are still in two separate pronuclei, and until these are joined no sure human potential exists. Much can still go wrong.

Egg plus sperm . . . Perhaps the decisive moment comes later, when the mother's and father's chromosomes intermingle. Shortly after this the cell divides, some twenty-four hours after the sperm first penetrated the outer membrane of the egg, and at that point its human potential might indeed be said to be established. But this stage is in fact no more decisive than any of its predecessors. In the fertilisation of an egg, be it human, fish or frog, all stages are necessary and all are interdependent.

Besides, even after this apparently final stage, the individual still is not fixed. An embryo requires two more days to switch on its genes and will never grow far unless it implants in its mother's womb. Furthermore, twins or triplets long implanted in their mothers exchange parts as they grow. They swap cells so that many become mixtures of the originals. One may die, and the survivor or survivors live on with its ghostly genetic memory, combinations of embryos that scientists call chimaeras. Identical twins or triplets further complicate the situation, for these may arise as many as fourteen days after the fertilisation process. So that even if a decisive moment were somehow established, it need not produce a single human being. And some embryos with Down's syndrome constantly change their disastrous inheritance, the unfortunate unwanted extra chromosome being found in fewer and fewer cells as the fetus develops.

Not that egg plus sperm are invariably needed to produce a living embryo. Unfertilised mouse eggs can turn into embryos if dipped in alcohol, or warmed or chilled, or given an electric shock. Embryonic life starts immediately, with unique sets of genes and chromosomes inherited from the mother only. Scientists call this parthenogenesis, and can generate hundreds of fatherless embryos in a couple of hours in any embryology laboratory. And what is possible for mice is almost certainly possible for humans. Indeed, given the scientific will (an important proviso!), the day of the fatherless human baby might not be far off.

Nature still is not finished with the absolutists. There are motherless embryos too, arising when all the mother's chromosomes are discarded. These embryos turn into grossly distorted fetuses called hydatidiform moles, huge masses of tissue in the womb that may even turn into a life-threatening cancer. The placenta, the organ that should nourish the embryo, explodes into growth as the fetus decays: it becomes hugely swollen, disfiguring the mother, and it must be removed to save her from serious injury or death.

To sum up, basing any embryological argument, or ethical decision, or legal prohibition upon the moment of fertilisation is dangerously simplistic. No such moment exists.

Furthermore, to wish that it did seems to me to deny the fundamental wholeness and beauty of creation.

Life is continuous. It is not the opposite of death — it is a tender, ever-changing thread, a delicate link between the generations. It has no stop-watch beginning, and its end returns it to the whole biomass of our planet. Embryology therefore, which is about life, is about movement: it is about the gradual unfolding as egg and spermatozoa become embryo, fetus, child and adult, and as adults form still

further eggs and spermatozoa. Spermatozoa and unfertilised eggs are alive, as alive as embryos and fetuses
– and incidentally should be protected at least as watchfully
as those, since nature itself could become perverted if
genetic engineers were recklessly to introduce new genes
into them.

What this discussion of an embryo's beginnings finally
tells us, therefore, is that reverence for the whole is needed,
reverence for life itself, and that our unique human-ness will
be defended with wisdom only if this basic fact is
understood.

# The Human Embryo
# 2. Donation: spermatozoa, eggs and embryos

In today's society, mothers and fathers might not be what
they seem. Children can now be conceived within marriage
even if a man has no spermatozoa and his wife no eggs. The
method is simple: sperm or egg can be donated from one
person to another, and embryos from one couple to
another. So parents might not be genetically related at all to
their growing family.

Sperm donation is hardly a new technique. When the
donor spermatozoa can, of course, reach the egg as a result
of coitus, this is the natural reproductive process. But
spermatozoa can also be introduced to the egg artificially,
either into the womb via the vagina, or in a culture dish.
Donor insemination has been possible since the end of the
eighteenth century, following the first artificial insemination by John Hunter, a British scientist. When semen is
required from male animals for purposes of artificial
insemination it is usually obtained by employing a receptacle in the shape and at the temperature of a vagina during

the natural mating process, but from humans the spermatozoa are produced by means of masturbation. Recent deep freezing techniques have enabled spermatozoa to be kept without harm for very long periods, and substantial sperm banks exist in many parts of the world.

The possibility that eggs might be donated from one woman to another arose only some twenty years ago, when I first ripened eggs outside the body, in a culture medium, but it wasn't really practised until the 1970s, when laparoscopy enabled Patrick to pluck already ripened eggs from human ovaries.

Since the first eggs were in fact fertilised in vitro with the husbands' spermatozoa and replaced in their mothers for attempts at IVF pregnancies, the procedure was done entirely within marriage, and did not involve egg donation. Eggs from another woman could easily have been used, however, and the resulting embryo replaced in the wife: this would have been egg donation.

Alternatively, an egg could have been fertilised by donated sperm and placed in the womb of yet another woman, neither the original donor nor the man's wife. This would have been embryo donation.

Finally, if the child resulting from an egg or embryo donation were delivered and then returned to the care of its genetic mother, the procedure would have been surrogate mothering.

There is an overwhelming medical case for sperm, egg and embryo donation. Some men produce too few spermatozoa to bring about conception – occasionally none at all – and this is a defect that remains incurable, the testes being just far too complicated for modern medicine. If these men and their wives want children genetically related to at least one of them, sperm donation is the only answer. Some women's ovaries are excised for medical reasons, or their egg supply simply runs out while they are still young, so that they face a premature menopause. Since these women are often able to gestate an egg fertilised by their husband, egg donation for them can be the perfect answer to childlessness. Then again, one or other member of a couple, or sometimes both, may carry a crippling genetic disease such as haemophilia, and these will need a sperm, an egg, or an embryo from a donor if they are to experience any part of the joy of child-bearing and rearing.

It is usual for a doctor, with their consent, to choose the donor, but some couples take the matter into their own hands; there is a national semen bank in France, the donors being family men of known fertility and genetics who consult their family about donation first, and there are banks in America that offer clients sperm from men of proven athletic ability or high IQ — these are presumably patronised by couples who mistakenly believe that the children of such fathers can be relied upon to be similarly endowed. Much more sensible are the rhesus-negative wives of rhesus-positive husbands, for example, who, fearing that their children will suffer from haemolytic disease, have quietly and privately found a rhesus-negative man to father their children, thus sparing them all chance of the disease.

Deciding between the acceptance of donated sperm, egg or embryo and adoption (which is becoming increasingly difficult to organise these days) can be very difficult and painful for a couple. They have to come to terms with their infertility, and accept that their child will not be biologically related to one or both of them, and they need time, good counselling, and lots of sympathy as they make their decision. Raising the child as their own is a lifelong commitment, agreement as to what the child is to be told has to be reached (and kept to!), and they are encouraged to think deeply before embarking on it. Even so, a thousand such babies are born each year in Britain, mostly from donor insemination, and ten times more in the USA.

Donor insemination wins few points for scientific or medical subtlety. Usually a doctor places the semen in the woman's vagina, but she can inseminate herself if she chooses. Insemination is more reliably successful if it is timed to coincide with ovulation, or if washed spermatozoa are injected directly into the womb, but such sophistications are not usually necessary. It can be performed confidentially and quickly, at a clinic on the way to work or to the shops, and has a high success rate.

Egg and embryo donation are more complex, and rarer. The number of women with no eggs, who are still youthful enough to carry fetuses, is not large. Some have no ovaries, others use up their egg store, and many need help because their menstrual cycles don't begin at puberty, or their menstrual rhythm fades in their teens or twenties – the premature menopause I have already mentioned. In this connection, employing a well-known method of giving hormones that establish artificial cycles in women at the natural menopause and thus help them over this difficult period, an Australian medical team has transferred an embryo to a young woman with a premature menopause during such an artificial cycle, and has begun a successful pregnancy. It was a novel piece of work.

Some clinics now practise egg donation on a fairly regular basis. They may recruit donors or they may take a short cut by requesting two or three extra eggs from patients already attending for their own IVF. Those women with more than nine or ten are asked to donate two or three, an easy practice in a busy clinic where patients come every day of the week and there is a regular supply of eggs. Easy but dangerous, since such donors and recipients are too briefly in the clinic for adequate counselling on the emotional complexities of donation. They have no time to consider its deeper implications, while the mystery and generosity involved in giving away such an intimate potential for life spurs them on. Predictably, therefore, donors aren't always happy with their decision afterwards.

Donating eggs may be little different ethically from donating spermatozoa, and indeed many women take the fate of their eggs as lightly as most men take the fate of their sperm. (The first request to an ethical committee for egg donation was made in Oldham in 1977: 'Project No. 2, submitted by Mr P.C. Steptoe . . . It is proposed to carry out transfer of an oöcyte from a volunteer donor fertilised by the recipient husband's spermatozoa.' Approval was granted, subject to genetic screening and the prospective parents' agreement to consider the child as their own, and we made one attempt which unfortunately failed.) Practical difficulties exist in egg donation however. It is much harder to conceal the egg donor's identity. She receives hormone injections and her follicles are scanned regularly, and it is even possible that she may be in the same hospital as the recipient as she waits to give her eggs away. This is less likely today, now that eggs and embryos can be deep-frozen, for the recipient may attend for her IVF weeks or months later.

The situation of a woman receiving donated eggs is emotionally easier than that of a husband agreeing to a sperm donation. An egg recipient gestates the fetus, from a few days after fertilisation by her husband until delivery, and thus both she and her husband retain an important biological role in 'making' the child. In contrast, the husband in a donor insemination plays no genuinely biological part in the child's conception or birth. Such emotional nuances may seem trivial, but they can cause great unhappiness if they are not foreseen and dealt with in advance.

For a woman, egg and embryo donation must be recognised as profoundly radical, involving a fundamental change in human affairs, for they break the most atavistic link of all, that between a mother and her child. Even if, as in egg donation, the embryo is fertilised by her husband, the recipient bears a child totally unrelated to her. She is the uterine mother, but a genetic onlooker, and she may feel this alien-ness very keenly. For this reason some couples prefer embryo donation, in which the child is related genetically to neither, for then at least they share the same lack of family relationship with it.

The embryos used for donation may be grown in vitro after laparoscopy or ultrasound, but this is no longer necessary: they can now be flushed by lavage unharmed from the donor's womb, on the fifth day after she has had intercourse or artificial insemination. Lavage was pioneered in Chile some twenty years ago and has now been repeated in the USA. It is less traumatic, perhaps, than laparoscopy and it can be performed repeatedly on the same volunteer — the only serious risk being that she may become pregnant in the unlikely event that all of her fertilised eggs are not flushed out. Physicians specialising in embryo donation in Los Angeles have recruited several donors and repeatedly flush cleaving embryos, morulae and blastocysts from them, using these to establish pregnancies in women with no eggs of their own. Some doctors fear, though, that an embryo might be washed into the donor's oviduct, to form a dangerous ectopic pregnancy.

Another donation procedure, one that some people consider even more radical, is that of surrogate mother-hood, in which the embryo is gestated by an unrelated woman — usually for money, sometimes for love — and the child is then returned at birth to its genetic parents. This procedure is medically straightforward, but its moral, legal and political implications are complex, and I devote an entire chapter to it later in this book.

One further (but non-medical) solution to intractable infertility deserves mention. I myself had never heard of child donation until the early 1970s when, seated round a family dinner table in a country far from Britain, I was astonished to hear my host tell of his own experiences.

'My brother was infertile, you see, even after years of trying for a child. Meanwhile, my wife and I had one, two, three, without any difficulty. My brother and his wife were very unhappy, so we conceived two more children, just for them to have as their own. There was no question of contracts or payments — it was our duty, and we did it. We have all been very happy, and our kinship is even closer than before as our two families grow up side-by-side, completely unaware of their true relationship . . .'

This tale at the dinner table seemed so admirably

straightforward, generous, and simple. Perhaps that distant country had fewer legal controls than mine, but its ancient wisdom clearly reached deeper into essential ethical truth. So when I eventually got back to Oldham, I couldn't resist telling the story to a small group of doctors, one of them a grizzled old pathologist.

There was an unimpressed pause after I finished.

'Your tale doesn't surprise me,' the pathologist said. 'You may know a lot about reproduction, Dr Edwards, but you obviously don't know much about people. I've heard many a tale like that from around here in Lancashire. In fact, they do it all the time in Rochdale!'

# The Human Embryo
# 3. Embryos in cold store

Improvements in deep freezing methods with various cells and tissues in the 1940s, made the eventual freezing of human embryos inevitable. The technique began with animal embryos, first a few mouse embryos, but soon thousands of cattle grazing in the summer fields had spent part of their embryonic life at temperatures as low as $-196°C$, their growth arrested until the magic moment of thawing. Scientists around the world then extended their studies from animal to human embryos, and were eventually successful.

Newspaper columnists called the children resulting from thawed-out embryos *Ice Babies*, or *Frosties*. They made the headlines for a while, and their births seemed an astonishing achievement, the creation of suspended life. Now human embryos could be stored virtually indefinitely, providing mankind with a bizarre foothold in the future.

They attracted mass attention for a few months, but the readers and viewers soon became accustomed to them.

Today it is an accepted commonplace — so quickly do we come to terms with technological progress — that thousands of human embryos are kept frozen in suspended animation in banks around the world. The containers are specially designed, far more sophisticated than the familiar kitchen freezer, and at the unimaginable low temperatures within them all the biochemistry of life simply ceases. The actual freezing process is extremely delicate, as is the thawing-out stage, but the intermediate period is only a matter of efficient refrigeration.

The basic idea is hardly new — the notion of freezing spermatozoa was proposed as long ago as 1850, by an Italian scientist, Mantegazza. He predicted that the semen from farm animals would one day be frozen and transported over long distances for subsequent artificial insemination. He also saw that men killed on the battlefield would similarly, but posthumously, be able to produce legitimate offspring. The man had amazing foresight! Especially since the temperatures low enough to store spermatozoa did not become available for another forty years.

Eighty years passed, in fact, before American and French scientists reopened Mantegazza's work, and his dream became reality in 1949, when three British researchers, A.U. Smith, C. Polge and A.S. Parkes, froze non-human spermatozoa in liquid nitrogen, and showed that they remained fertile. The secret of their success lay in establishing the right conditions during freezing. At the low temperatures necessary the structure of spermatozoa changes as their biochemistry slows down, and dangerous gases become soluble, threatening their survival. Ice forms also, removing water, so that the suspending solutions are concentrated and become toxic. But it was found that chemicals such as glycerol or dimethysulphoxide, DMSO for short, protected the spermatozoa as they froze, thus enabling many to survive. Other additives helped too, in particular the yolk of a fresh hen's egg.

Research had already turned to human spermatozoa, and

pioneering work was done by Landrum B. Shettles in America. Human sperm were found to be less cooperative, but combinations of the same preservatives worked in the end. Many samples were soon in store, from donors of known characteristics, their race, complexion, height and weight carefully recorded. Specialised centres provided ampoules to clients, and a national service was established in France.

It was just as Mantegazza had predicted. Once his semen was frozen, a husband could be away at war, or abroad on business, and still conceive a child, and some widows were indeed able to bear their husbands' children long after the men were dead, by means of their frozen semen.

Marginally infertile men may be helped too, by conserving their restricted number of gametes and accumulating them over several weeks. Some men have a personal sperm bank established before they are exposed to X-rays to treat their cancer, or to drugs that might destroy their chances of fatherhood. Although success rates do vary from man to man, the records of the French central registry have shown that storing semen is simple and effective.

Success with spermatozoa inevitably led cryobiologists – researchers into the effects of very low temperatures on living organisms – to work on the freezing of eggs and embryos. In the early 1970s a British scientist, David Whittingham, claimed to have frozen mouse embryos which developed normally after being thawed and placed in recipient females. Although his work was not fully accepted it provided a useful basis for the freezing of human embryos, and later – collaborating now with two American scientists, Leibo and Mazur – Whittingham was able to clarify the correct conditions for the slow freezing and subsequent thawing of mouse embryos.

Glycerol and DMSO were successful again, helping the embryos to reach very low temperatures virtually unharmed, and enabling them to be thawed again simply by plunging the vial containing them into warm water. It

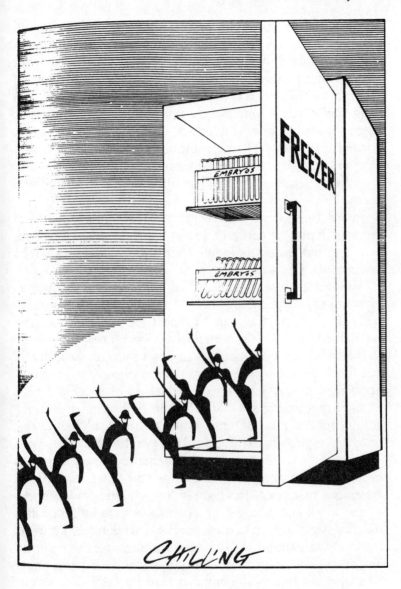

CHILLING

seemed that mouse embryos at all stages could be stored indefinitely, whether 4-cell, 8-cell, or blastocysts. After a year, and again at yearly intervals, a dozen or so were thawed and examined and a few were damaged beyond recognition. Others survived with only half of their original cells, while many were intact, almost as new, yet most of them, perfect and imperfect, implanted and grew successfully in foster mothers – in their own mothers' daughters and even their grand-daughters – and the offspring were normal. The implications for man were plain.

In no time at all the technique was applied to farm animals. Banks of cattle embryos were frozen and stored, awaiting the magic moment when they would be thawed and replaced in a recipient cow.

The science of freezing living organisms is known as cryobiology. Cryobiologists try to freeze and revive many sorts of living matter, but to date their success has been restricted to the simplest organisms. A venturesome few try to freeze whole human bodies in an attempt to cheat death, but this technique, known as cryonics, is practised more in hope than in any very firm expectation of success.

The cryobiologist's skill lies in choosing the right conditions and rates of temperature change for freezing and thawing, especially in the crucial temperature band between $-36$ and $-40°C$ during which damage is most likely to occur, and the optimum conditions still remain uncertain. Ingenious machinery has been invented. One device works by puffing liquid nitrogen at a controlled rate into a central freezing well, with much clicking and winking of lights as the gas swirls round vials of embryos, coaxing them gently into suspended animation. Another machine also uses liquid nitrogen, but lowers the embryo vials by very slow stages into its freezing chamber.

I myself had decided to try freezing human eggs and embryos in Oldham back in 1977, driven by our lack of pregnancies in IVF patients. With this in mind I delivered a paper at the first conference ever to discuss the matter: 'The storage of human preimplantation embryos at low temperatures could be invaluable . . . for the alleviation of infertility and possibly to avoid genetic defects in children.' (R.G. Edwards and P.C. Steptoe. *The Freezing of Mammalian Embryos*, Ciba Foundation Symposium, Elsevier, Amsterdam, 1977.)

Some of my colleagues expressed reservations: there might be long-term genetic consequences from freezing and I was expecting too much of cryobiology. Other speakers were on my side, quoting the extensive evidence already available from work on animal embryos.

I decided there was medical and scientific justification for going ahead. The next stage was for Patrick to submit an application to his hospital ethical committee for permission to carry out the procedure. Thus, in an uninspiring corner of Lancashire, the Oldham and District General Hospital became the first medical authority in the world in 1977 to assess and give ethical judgment on the freezing of human embryos.

'Project No. 2, submitted by Mr P.C. Steptoe.

'Proposal to explore the storage and re-implantation of embryos in order to overcome the problems of implantation.

'Embryos to be obtained after in-vitro fertilisation of oöcytes with patients with absent or hopelessly diseased tubes . . . High failure rate of bringing about successful implantation in the recovery indicates we should store the embryos and replant them in a subsequent cycle . . .

'AGREED, subject to the following: (i) that an independent witness checks the embryos; (ii) that the case notes should be kept for longer than the statutory period: these cases would require longer follow-up.'

Jean and I got to work. The first embryos were sent from Oldham to David Whittingham for freezing in London – by courtesy of British Railways, and the guards on the Manchester–London expresses can have had no idea of the

momentous contents of the packages they handled for us so
efficiently! David was optimistic — after freezing and
thawing the embryos still seemed to be in very reasonable
condition. Encouraged, we were able later to install a
freezing machine of our own in Oldham, to wink and click
and puff day and night in its own little room.

'It huffed endlessly, pumping a bitterly cold gas into its
freezing chamber, one puff at a time, blinking its green light
each time it exhaled . . . Opening a door at night, peering
into the dark room, the night nurses must have taken a step
backwards when confronted by this hissing, winking green
light contraption that pumped out clouds of gas.' (*A Matter
of Life*, R.G. Edwards and P.C. Steptoe, Hutchinson, London,
1980.)

Many of the frozen eggs and embryos looked good on
thawing, with cells still alive and active, a good sign for
further growth. If we had persevered with our experiments
for a little longer we might well have opened up the whole
field of human cryobiology there and then, but that was the
time when Lesley Brown successfully implanted one of her
own fresh embryos, and it became more important for us to
concentrate on in-vitro fertilisation by this means.

Someone else was bound to freeze and successfully thaw
human embryos, so we watched with interest as scientists in
the Netherlands and Australia published their research
findings. Quickest to achieve success was a team led by
Alan Trounson at Monash University in Melbourne. In
1982, using DMSO to freeze a cleaving embryo, they later
established a pregnancy with the thawed embryo, but
unfortunately it aborted.

Then reports began to circulate that Gerard Zeilmaker,
working in the Netherlands, had established a pregnancy
with an embryo that had previously been frozen. He was
cautious about making a firm announcement, however,
even though identical twins were born of the pregnancy,
because the case was not entirely straightforward. One
cause for doubt was that the couple concerned, although

long infertile, were seemingly healthy and capable of reproduction, so that they might in fact have conceived in the normal way. It was also difficult to explain how their twins could have resulted from the replacement of a single thawed embryo.

Such doubts have faded with time and new knowledge. Zeilmaker's couple was certainly infertile – they have failed to conceive naturally ever since, despite repeated efforts. Their embryo must have divided into twins, as many do in women who have been given fertility drugs, probably because its membrane was hardened, splitting the blastocyst in two. Many other identical twins have arisen like this, after in-vitro fertilisation or when ovarian stimulants are given to women. No, Zeilmaker's twins almost certainly deserve to be regarded as the first children ever of an embryo conceived in vitro and then deep-frozen and, to his credit, Alan Trounson accepts this conclusion.

Zeilmaker's caution resulted in an Australian baby being awarded that distinction. In April, 1984, the Melbourne team's second pregnancy was successful.

'The world's first deep-freeze baby.' (The *Daily Mail*, 11 April 1984)

'First frozen-embryo birth.' (*The Times*, 12 April 1984.) 'The Melbourne team has frozen 230 embryos, 40 of which have been thawed. Of these, 23 survived and were transferred . . . The birth . . . could be matched in Britain within two years.'

*The Times* was out of date! We were hard at work in Bourn Hall by then after an enforced delay while several ethical groups decided on their attitudes to freezing, and our first frozen-embryo baby was born only a matter of weeks after the one in Melbourne. But we certainly weren't able to match the next item of frozen-embryo news to come out of Australia.

In June 1984, a Mr and Mrs Rios, the parents of two embryos they had had frozen, were killed in a plane crash. They died intestate, so that their fortune was to be inherited either by a distant relative or – just possibly – by one or both of the embryos, should they be successfully implanted and produce a child or children.

The legal situation was complex, the medical situation rather less so. Carl Wood, the head of the Australian IVF team, was reported as saying: 'They are unlikely to survive any attempt to implant them in a womb because the techniques used at the time they were frozen were not as good as they are now.'

Even so, what should be done with them?

'Test-tube embryos orphaned.' (The *Daily Telegraph*, 18 June 1984)

Eventually the Australian Minister of Health for the State of Victoria, who had been appointed the embryos' legal guardian, obtained special legislation: they could be donated to any couple that was agreeable, but any child or children born as a result would not inherit the natural parents' estate. It was a wise decision, and the fuss quickly died down.

By now, of course, ice babies themselves are rarely news. Sometimes there are charges, never substantiated, of an international trade in frozen embryos. Then again, two frozen Bourn Hall twins were born eighteen months apart, so a controversy grew up as to whether they were twins or not. And there are different opinions on how long to store embryos for a couple, whether they should only be replaced in the wife or donated to someone else, or replaced in the mother or the father's new wife following a divorce or if one or both parents died. And, of course, the inevitable doubts as the banks of frozen embryos multiplied, with thousands in store. But by now one hundred or more babies must have been born, mostly at Bourn Hall, in Melbourne and in France. One hundred precious babies who have spent a year or more of their embryonic lives at $-196°C$. Women with cancer or other diseases requiring chemotherapy which may well, as a side effect, destroy their ovaries, now have the promise of egg banks, just as the men have sperm banks, and therefore the chance later, when they are cured, of handing on the miracle of their own lives to their children.

The old freezing method, using a slow decline in temperature by means of gradually increasing exposure to liquid nitrogen, will almost certainly soon be obsolete. High concentrations of DMSO in the preservative solution seem to make very rapid freezing and thawing possible. And even simpler techniques are in sight: vitrification using a mixture of chemicals, or desiccation, in which the water is extracted before the freezing process begins. And a different cryopreservative has been used in Paris: propanediol appears to enable fertilised eggs and cleaving embryos to be stored virtually without damage. Success rates using such embryos have risen dramatically, and many clinics are adopting the method.

All stages of human embryonic life are now in the deep freeze, banked in their thousands across Europe, Australia and North and South America. Ice babies have conclusively arrived.

In 1985 the *Daily Mail* gave a headline to the first birthday of one of them: 'The ice baby. Glow of love for Gregory, the deep freeze baby'.

Gregory's second birthday slipped past without comment.

# The Human Embryo
# 4. Research on embryos

If there are disagreements about the donation or freezing of human embryos, far greater passions are aroused about the need to carry out research on them. Everyone knows in principle that medical advances are built on scientific research, but the necessity or otherwise for experiments on human embryos sparks the most intense argument, as fears arise about tailor-made babies, or clones, or cyborgs, or some other nightmarish fancy.

The trouble really started way back in the 1930s, by courtesy of the brilliant Aldous Huxley. In his novel, *Brave New World*, his Director of Hatcheries and Conditioning spoke thus: '"These," he waved his hand, "are the incubators . . . The week's supply of ova. Kept at blood heat; whereas the male gametes" – and here he opened another door – "they have to be kept at thirty-five instead of thirty-seven."' He went on to describe how the Alphas and Betas remained until definitely bottled, while the Gammas, Deltas and Epsilons were brought out again after only thirty-six hours . . . to bud, and proliferate into ninety-six perfectly formed embryos: '"Identical twins – but not in piddling two and threes . . . by dozens, scores at a time, thousands . . . Standard men and women; in uniform batches."'

Admittedly some of Huxley's notions have come true. Fifty ova can now be collected from a human ovary. This is a modest figure compared with his thousands, yet his ideas still grip prophets of doom more than any other science fiction, as the numbers of human embryos growing in vitro rise year by year, and as his fellow writers whip up forebodings dire enough to alarm even the most phlegmatic science watcher. Whatever today's embryologists may do, Frankenstein or Faust or Jekyll will have foreshadowed, looming over every biological debate. They leave science far behind – and in many cases it doesn't even want to catch up.

Cloning, as I have already mentioned, is a case in point. Although no human embryologist working seriously in the field today has any great interest in it, cloning remains one of the favourite bugaboos for the cheap press and the writers of science horror stories.

Invented by two American scientists twenty years ago, the word *cloning* initially described studies on frogs, in which a nucleus from an adult was injected into an enucleate egg, and the resulting embryo – or at least the very small proportion of the eggs that developed into embryos – grew up into carbon copies of the donor. So far, cloning can be done only very modestly in mammals, by transferring a nucleus from a morula or blastocyst to a mouse egg, and even then the resulting embryos are rare. And certainly nobody seems to be interested in trying it with human embryos. Cloning might also mean something rather different today. A 2-cell egg can now be divided into two embryos – into identical twins, two clones – or a 4-cell embryo into identical quadruplets. This can be done fairly easily in animals, and it might one day be attempted in humans, to raise the chances of a pregnancy by replacing two embryos instead of one. The two half-embryos might grow well, because one-half of the cells in a frozen embryo might be destroyed yet it can grow to a baby when thawed and replaced in its mother.

In fact, of course, despite all the horror stories, most people connect embryo research with the early diagnosis or treatment of crippling diseases and therefore will concede, if pressed, that such research has been, and will continue to be, of great material benefit to humanity. None of the current developments in in-vitro fertilisation, either, would have been possible without it.

Back in 1968 detailed embryo research had been needed in Oldham before we could locate eggs ripening naturally in their mothers' ovaries and extract them, and before we could discover the solutions that would support fertilisation and ensure normal growth until the embryo's careful return to its mother.

I well remember the day, a year or so later, when I sat with Patrick in his office in the Oldham and District General Hospital. We were both enormously excited, for we had just seen for ourselves through a microscope four beautiful human blastocysts, the first ever grown in culture. They seemed outwardly perfect, but we had yet to be certain of their inner structure.

'"What are we going to do with them?" Patrick asked.

"We're going to flatten them, to check their chromosomes," I replied.

"So what do I tell my patients?" Patrick insisted.

"I've got to see that the cell nuclei and the chromosomes are good," I said. "We will be able to explain to them that we have taken another step forward."' (*A Matter of Life*, Edwards and Steptoe.)

Was this the right decision? The right decision for Patrick's patients, or the right decision for science? It was a fair decision, but another might have been better. Those blastocysts could have been replaced in their mother's womb rather than used as research material. But then, imagine the public outcry if, as a result of my not checking their nuclei and chromosomes, the first child born of IVF had been defective! Our work would have been stopped dead. Without research on those early embryos there would have been no test-tube babies for the infertile, not even now, twenty years later.

It must be said, here at the very outset, that embryo research often results in the destruction of these microscopic living organisms. An embryo removed from its culture fluid dies very quickly. Many kinds of in-vitro examination also damage embryos so that they no longer develop. Embryos that are either dead or seriously deformed are destroyed: incinerated with other laboratory waste as often as not. Some of these, if returned carefully to a woman's womb, might possibly have developed into human beings, possibly into malformed human beings. There are rights and wrongs to this, and I will discuss them later.

Undeniably, research on human embryos is still desperately needed, and for many purposes. First of all, to clarify the causes of human genetic disasters in the hope of averting them. Research on ripening eggs, for example, at the moment when the chromosomes — twenty-three in normal conditions — are reorganising themselves before ovulation.

I wrote about this in *A Matter of Life*: 'Chromosomes . . . moved like soldiers through a prepared drill. First they marched to the centre of the egg, then out to the periphery. Next they separated into two . . . as they glided along the spindle . . . one half marched out of the egg for ever . . . The purpose . . . was to prepare the egg for fertilisation, and the precision of it all . . . was breath-taking.' I first watched these events in mouse eggs thirty years ago. I see them now regularly in human eggs, and I marvel still.

One tiny mistake at this moment and the embryo inherits an extra chromosome, perhaps more, which will play havoc with its growth. Just one mistake, and children are born to abnormal sexual development, or with Down's syndrome or other distressing diseases, incurable and overwhelming obstacles to normal growth.

Why do some chromosomes miss their way? One possibility is that the error occurred back when the eggs themselves were forming in their mother's ovary, when she was herself a fetus. If so, then sadly they can never be recognised in the adult woman, among the hundreds of thousands of eggs she has, so the anomaly can never be avoided. This would be bad news, but far better we know it rather than live in false hopes.

Some malformed embryos are even worse. They have sixty-nine chromosomes and these arise as two sper-matozoa drive into an egg, adding their forty-six chromo-somes to its twenty-three. These eggs have three pronuclei, as in the case of Mrs Dawson's tenth egg, and have no chance at all of developing normally. It would be possible to remove one pronucleus, which would revert the egg to normal, and I'm often tempted to do so. But we know too little: such heroic surgery might make matters even worse in some way we don't yet understand, causing still greater damage to the embryo's future growth.

Sometimes the mother passes her forty-six chromosomes to her embryo. Most of the resulting fetuses abort naturally, but a few form severely abnormal children, doomed to a year or two of wretched life. A few human embryos have more chromosomes still, ninety-two or even more, and indeed embryos carrying imbalanced chromosomes form a regular and distressing part of our inheritance. Many die in the mother before she knows she's pregnant, and virtually all the rest decay from three to six months later, a bitter disappointment just as she is beginning to anticipate a happy delivery. But occasionally one survives, to be born tragically impaired.

Admittedly, research on embryos will not help those children already afflicted. But one in five embryos has a chromosomal error, perhaps more, and only research on human eggs, sperm and embryos will identify the origins of such errors. There is no other way, none at all, and until we understand the origins we can do nothing to prevent them. Perhaps we won't be able to even then, but surely we should try?

Secondly, research is needed to improve fertilisation rates. Interestingly, Huxley writes of IVF in his novel *Brave New World* with impressive accuracy as his Director of Hatcheries and Conditioning describes how 'eggs . . . were inspected for anomalies, counted and transferred to a porous receptacle; how . . . this receptacle was immersed in a warm bouillon containing free-swimming spermatozoa — at a minimum concentration of one hundred thousand per cubic centimetre . . .'

Compare this with our words in the *British Journal of Obstetrics and Gynaecology* almost fifty years later: 'Oöcytes were transferred into suspensions of spermatozoa held in microdrops. The concentrations of spermatozoa ranged from under one hundred thousand to one million per cubic centimetre, depending upon the proportion of mobile spermatozoa in the ejaculate.'

Unfortunately, even in such huge quantities apparently healthy spermatozoa still often fail to penetrate the egg's outer membrane, and we do not yet know why. This is not mere scientific greed, curiosity for curiosity's sake. It might just be possible to physically inject a sperm into an egg, to help infertile men to conceive. In any case, not only can further research teach us how to help infertile men to fertilise their wife's eggs, but the reverse may also apply: such research may also teach us how to develop new contraceptive techniques, sparing men and women the intrusiveness of present methods.

Thirdly, research is needed to discover why the cells of some human embryos disintegrate, and why some stop growing. They display these signs of death almost as soon as they begin their short, forlorn lives, and we see them in embryo flushed naturally from their mother's wombs, as well as those in our culture fluids. Perhaps their chromosomes are wrong, perhaps fertilisation was too late, perhaps they suffered a metabolic shock. Or perhaps their immediate surroundings failed them, their environment. They must be kept neither too hot nor too cold, and be exposed neither to excesses of acid or of alkali. They need food, and they need oxygen – embryos eat and respire just as we do, except that their diet is rather more limited, consisting initially of a simple chemical called pyruvate, and then a sugar, glucose, a little later.

We already know how much they consume, and how their diet changes as they grow. We worked with Henry Leese, using his methods to meticulously measure the diets of human embryos, and found how some consumed more than others. If these could be shown to be the rare 15 per cent able to implant in their mothers, then measuring an embryo's appetite would promise identifying those with the best chance of surviving and even some with genetic diseases affecting their metabolism. Progress in this area has been very slow. Today an embryologist usually has plenty of developing eggs to choose from, but no proven way of making his choice, and he knows that only 15 per cent will establish pregnancies. Back in Oldham, when Louise Brown was born and we were working on a shoestring, the figure for established pregnancies was only very slightly less – around 12.5 per cent.

Fourthly, research is needed in order to discover when and how embryos synthesise their large molecules of inheritance, their DNA, and their vast variety of proteins and enzymes. Such molecules confer structure and specificity on their cells: they make each man or woman unique, and their mechanisms have philosophical as well as medical implications. We are only grown-up embryos, you and I, so it behoves us to try to understand these forces shaping our destiny.

This line of research may well shed light on other questions, such as that of cancer. In this connection the biochemist, R. Williamson, points out: 'It is thought that there are about a hundred thousand coding genes in the human genome, although only one-tenth of these are expressed in most tissues. A higher proportion are expressed in the early mammalian embryo . . . Embryonic gene expression and its control are of course also related to the problem of cancer, in which cells often revert to a fetal protein pattern.'

In other words, a proper understanding of the way early fetal cells develop could well provide vital insights into the development of cancerous cells (which are very similar), and therefore into therapies for their suppression.

Research into fetal DNA also holds the promise of new clinical breakthroughs. For one thing, fetuses stricken with mental or physical disabilities − at present not identified until ten weeks of gestation or even five months of pregnancy when their fluids or cells can be extracted and analysed − may well be able to be detected much sooner, in a cleaving embryo or blastocyst, while the entire organism is still a minute speck. The trauma of abortion could then be avoided if parents found the prospect of a severely handicapped child too hard for them to bear.

This is because research on rabbit blastocysts taught us, Richard Gardner and me, how to determine the sex of embryos using a few cells excised at a very early stage for diagnosis. Sexing human blastocysts by analysing their

DNA might be feasible, as we and others have shown, and replacing only female embryos in mothers known to be carrying certain hereditary conditions could greatly reduce the numbers of babies with haemophilia, muscular dystrophy and other disabling afflictions found almost entirely in males.

DNA amplification is a new and enormously powerful tool. Even the minute alterations caused by a single gene may be detected, by multiplying a thousandfold the tiny amount of DNA taken from an embryo and analysing its characteristics. One cell removed from an embryo might be enough, for American workers have done this with a single human spermatozoön. And if this were done with human embryos, then the blastocysts carrying crippling genes could be identified and flushed away, sparing patients the unhappiness of abortion following a much later diagnosis. Soon – within a year or two – it might be possible to identify those embryos suffering from muscular dystrophy, rather than having to choose female embryos to avoid the birth of babies with this genetic disorder.

This is not to say that all less-than-perfect fetuses must be averted, destroyed in their mothers' wombs or even before they get there. Every case, and every parent, makes his or her own rules. An author has spoken on this subject, not Aldous Huxley this time but Christopher Nolan, a severely spastic young man who describes his own view of life, his every word wrung from him letter by letter, with the help of a specially adapted word processor.

'. . . Tonight a crippled man is taking his place on the world literary stage. Tonight is my night for laughing, for crying tears of joy. But wait, my brothers hobble after me, hinting "What about silent us? Can we too have a voice?" . . . Imagine what I would have missed if the doctors had not revived me on that September day long ago . . .' His mother read this message on Nolan's behalf, when he was awarded the Whitbread Book of the Year prize in 1988, and it comes as an eloquent warning to doctors and counsellors in ante-natal clinics everywhere: each case is unique, and there are no simple answers.

And fifthly, research on human embryos is needed simply because, even at its most abstract, no line of study should be lightly abandoned. As science develops in its mysterious ways, what is abstract and rarified one day may very easily become urgently relevant the next. Chance discoveries have always been an essential part of scientific advance. Little did Alexander Fleming realise, when he noticed back in the 1920s that colonies of bacteria died in the vicinity of a certain fungus, that this chance observation would lead to a systematic study resulting in the discovery of penicillin and the introduction of antibiotics into medicine and their widespread use today.

Similarly, nothing we can learn about the secrets of early embryonic life, no matter how unplanned, is ever likely to go to waste. I remember well, for example, how we in Oldham allowed an embryo to grow in our culture medium beyond day five, and escape completely from its surrounding membrane. 'We watched it day by day with wonder. Monday, Tuesday, Wednesday, Thursday . . . more days of growth! The embryo was still a speck, but for me it represented . . . the actual moments when the foundations are being laid for the formation of the body's organs . . .' (*A Matter of Life*). Other embryos have grown for seven or eight days, then hesitated and seemed to die – we still don't know why – and on the eighth day have released a hormone into the culture medium. This turns out to have been a hormone typical of pregnancy, the first time such a compound had ever been recorded from an embryo grown in vitro, and it provided a vital clue about how embryos implant in their mothers. We had not expected such a result, we were not looking for it, but its consequences could be of benefit to literally thousands of women.

Not that all research is so unexceptionable. Some research is invasive: it changes the basic make-up of an embryo. We call it genetic engineering, and it was beyond

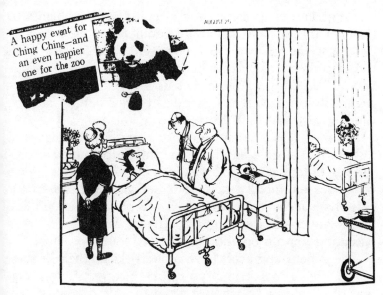

'Awfully sorry, Mrs Spinks. There seems to have been a dreadful mix-up at the test tube labs. . .'

even Huxley's wildest imaginings. At this very moment mice in laboratories all over the world are carrying genes that were injected when they were microscopic, newly-fertilised eggs – human genes perhaps, or cattle genes, alien substances which instruct their metabolisms to produce growth hormones, or antibodies, or novel medicines of one kind or another. These animals are called transgenics, and transgenic mice and pigs are tailored, for example, to produce the human growth hormone used in several child clinics, mostly in the USA.

In a field near Edinburgh, too, a flock of one hundred transgenic sheep are grazing. As *The Times* put it in September, 1987, 'Where gene-banks safely graze', for these sheep were capable of supplying enough human blood-clotting protein in their milk to treat all the haemophiliacs in Europe. No vast technological factory is needed – just a hundred sheep, their eggs manipulated in vitro, given human genes and a few other ingredients so that when they have grown into adults they produce that particular human protein and secrete it into their milk. Other proteins too, other hormones, can be made in this way. The US Patent Office has now given permission for such new forms of gene constructs to be patented, and for the animals that result to be patented also.

Commercialising new forms of animals is an alarming notion. It will give enormous incentive for purely profit-making organisations to break into the genetic inheritance of species and modify their fundamental characteristics, for entirely financial purposes. And it will of course imperil the free advance of science just a little more, as the laws of patenting impose on and curtail freedom of research.

The genetic engineers have other tricks up their sleeves. A cell from a mouse embryo can be incorporated into an unrelated mouse blastocyst, and its descendants will colonise major parts of the resulting offspring. Such donated cells might be able to repair a blastocyst ravaged by genetic disease, but for the moment the idea has not been pursued. Recently, however, one of my students, Peter Hollands, has used cells from mouse fetuses six or seven days old to colonise and repair young or adult mice suffering from anaemia or the effects of potentially lethal doses of X-rays — just like human beings who have been treated for cancer.

These donated cells are incredible: they are not rejected as adult grafts would be, and they sustain their recipients through full and healthy lives. Cells from rat embryos will even colonise mice, and human cells too. Cells such as these are known as stem cells, the foundations of the body's organs, and they can be obtained by growing blastocysts for a few days in vitro. American scientists have recently done similar work, using human blood cells to colonise mice.

Stem cells from human embryos may one day repair damaged children or adults, giving them new blood cells,

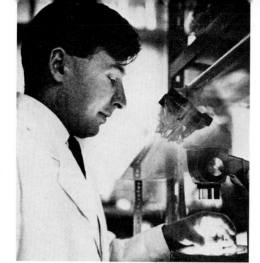

Working on animals
during my earlier years at
Cambridge.

Bourn Hall: the South
aspect of the ancient hall
with (left) part of the new
buildings.

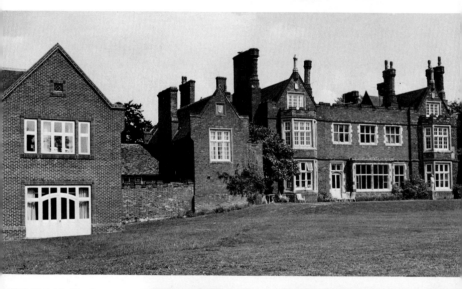

With Patrick Steptoe
during an intense
moment of public debate
at a press conference soon
after the birth of Louise
Brown, 1978.

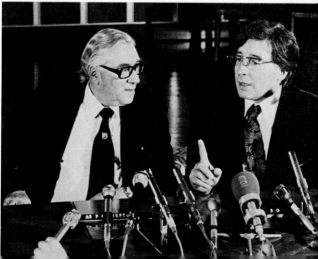

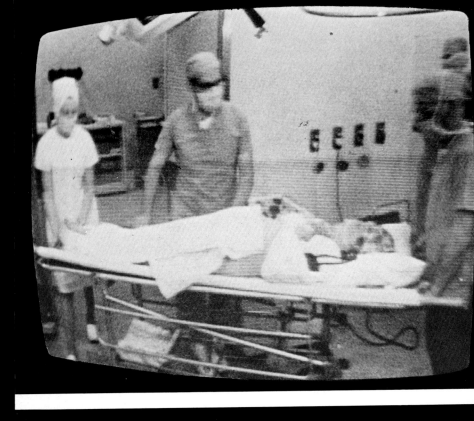
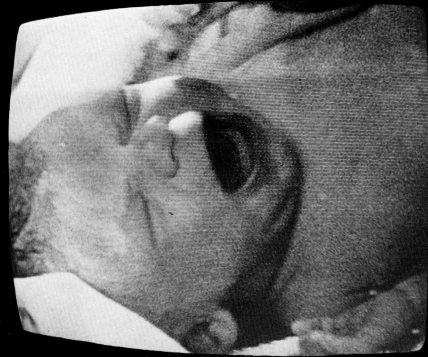

**Left:** Moments before Mrs Brown delivered her new baby – as captured on the hospital TV screen.

**Left below:** How the world first saw Louise.

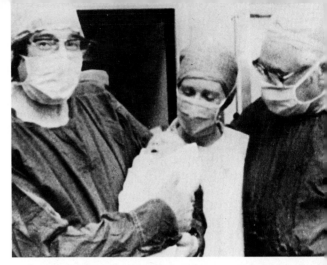

With Jean Purdy, Patrick and the new baby minutes after her delivery.

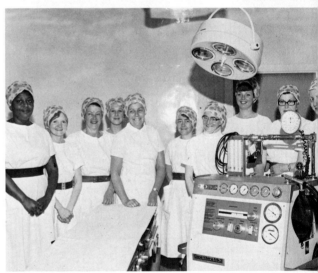

The sisters and nurses who worked on Louise's delivery at the Oldham and District General Hospital.

Louise with her parents shortly after the birth.

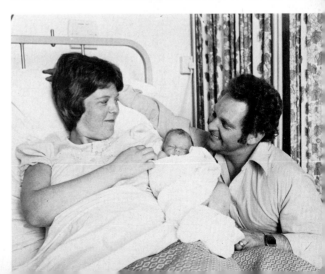

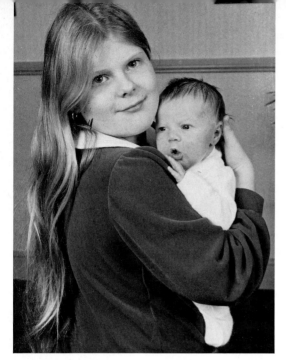

Louise now nine years old
holding the thousandth
baby conceived at Bourn
Hall.

Mr and Mrs Wright with
their 'twins' born 18
months apart. Were they
right in calling them
twins?

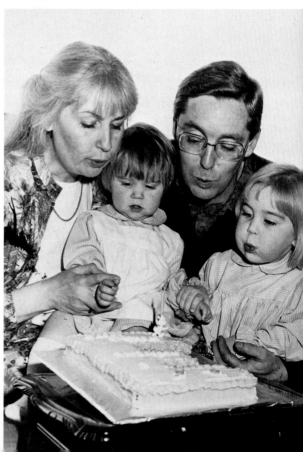

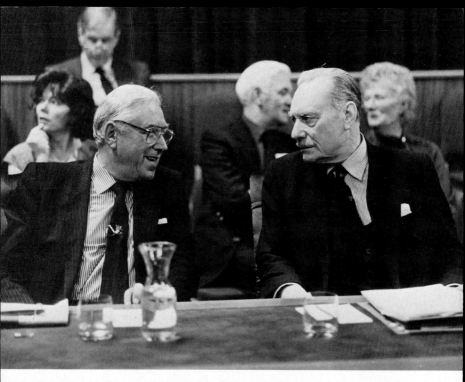

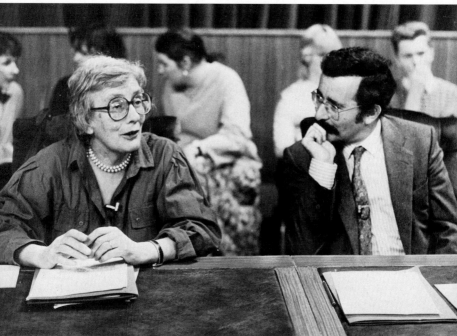

Patrick Steptoe looking light-hearted, while Enoch Powell seems to take matters more seriously during a discussion group in the late 1980s.

Mary Warnock and Robert Winstone share a quite moment.

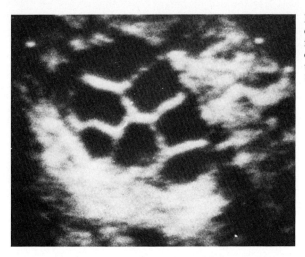

**Left:** Ultrasound scan of a human ovary showing seven large follicles, the largest with a diameter of 15 mm. Vaginal ultrasound was used.
⅓ natural size.

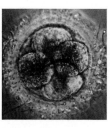

sperm lying outside egg membrane

**1:** Unfertilized egg with spermatozoa lying on its membrane.

A – egg membrane
B – polar body

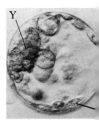

**2:** Spermatozoon just touching surface of egg, having forced its way through membrane. Its tail is still outside membrane, beating rapidly.

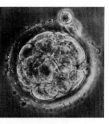

**3:** Two nuclei (pro nuclei), one from the sperm chromosome after entering the egg, one from the egg itself. If two spermatozoa enter the egg, 3 nuclei will lead to an abnormal embryo.

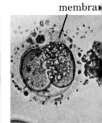

**4:** A 2-celled embryo the cells begin even and symmetrical. 3 hours after fertilization.

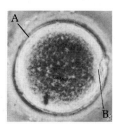

**5:** A 4-celled embryo 2 days after fertilization, the cells being even and symmetrical.

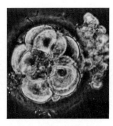

**6:** An 8-celled embryo 2½ days after fertilization. A clump of nurse cells from the ovary lie to the right of the embryo.

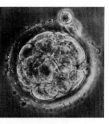

**7:** An embryo with 32 cells. 3½ days after fertilization.

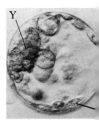

**8:** A blastocyst 4½ days after fertilization.
X – beginning of placental membrane that will protect the growing fetus.
Y – cells that will give rise to fetus and part of placenta.

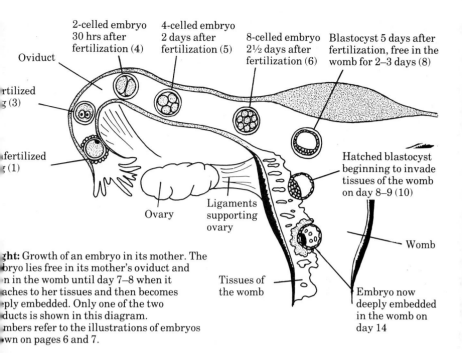

2-celled embryo
30 hrs after
fertilization (4)

4-celled embryo
2 days after
fertilization (5)

8-celled embryo
2½ days after
fertilization (6)

Blastocyst 5 days after
fertilization, free in the
womb for 2–3 days (8)

Oviduct

[ferti]lized
[egg] (3)

[un]fertilized
[egg] (1)

Hatched blastocyst
beginning to invade
tissues of the womb
on day 8–9 (10)

Womb

Ovary

Ligaments
supporting
ovary

Tissues of
the womb

Embryo now
deeply embedded
in the womb on
day 14

[Ri]ght: Growth of an embryo in its mother. The
[em]bryo lies free in its mother's oviduct and
[the]n in the womb until day 7–8 when it
[att]aches to her tissues and then becomes
[dee]ply embedded. Only one of the two
[ovi]ducts is shown in this diagram.
[Nu]mbers refer to the illustrations of embryos
[sho]wn on pages 6 and 7.

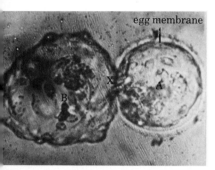

egg membrane

X

B

A

**Left:** (9) A blastocyst escaping (hatching) from
the egg membrane 6–7 days after fertilization.
Most of the embryo has escaped from A to B
through a small slit X which it has made in the
egg membrane, and is now growing outside.

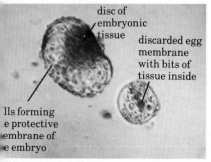

disc of
embryonic
tissue

discarded egg
membrane with bits of
tissue inside

[ce]lls forming
[th]e protective
[m]embrane of
[th]e embryo

[Ab]ove: (10) A 9-day blastocyst has now
[esc]aped completely from the egg membrane
[and] is expanding rapidly. It becomes attached
[to t]he womb just before this stage.

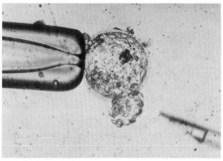

**Above:** Blastocyst held on a suction pipette
(on the left) and the small piece of extruded
tissues will be cut off with the glass knife (on
the right).

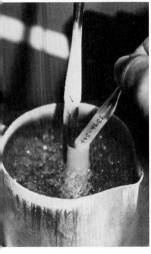

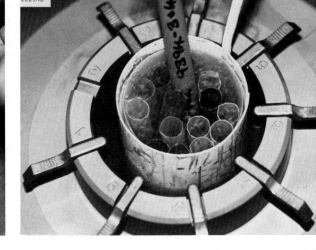

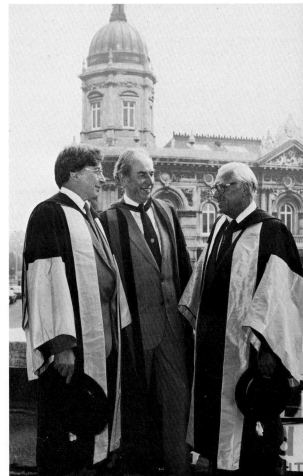

Another group of embryos, safe in their vial, goes into liquid nitrogen and is then placed in the storage container.

Official recognition of the value of in vitro fertilisation was long delayed, but finally D.Scs were awarded to both of us by Hull University in 1983. These were followed by a succession of other honours. Giving two D.Scs for one piece of research is highly unusual in any university.

new nerve cells, or new pancreatic cells, thus repairing anaemias, leukaemias, brain disorders, diabetes. Already in Sweden doctors are trying to repair brains, but with cells taken from much older fetuses, and other doctors in Mexico and Birmingham believe this technique will help to relieve the tragic symptoms of Parkinson's disease or Huntingdon's chorea. Also, blood cells from abortuses are given as therapy to men and women suffering from anti-cancer radiation or other blood deficiencies.

And how about those women with a premature menopause, those faced now with egg donation and hormone injections throughout their pregnancy for a low chance of success? Would an ovary graft from a fetus with its thousands and thousands of eggs restore their reproduction, or even extend it to much older years? Would cell donations like this help to alleviate the symptoms of the menopause? No one knows.

A future medicine can easily be imagined. Rows and rows of stem cells, deep-frozen, waiting to fight our cancers, to restore our paling blood or repair our fading brains. Stem cells able to mend a handicapped child while still in the womb, rather than aborting it as unsalvageable. Even stem cells with genes inserted into them, making them capable of tracking down and destroying a cancer, or possibly fighting the ravages of old age. Wild dreams, perhaps, but IVF itself would have been considered a wild dream forty years ago.

So research is needed – and research upon human embryos, since those of other species are too different to provide satisfactory models. 'How unique is human development?' the scientist Robert Williamson asked in a recent symposium. 'Obviously, all mammals share features of embryogenesis. However . . . some aspects of gene expression and determination are not common to all species. This is perhaps most apparent when we consider the brain and the nervous system . . .'

And where shall the human embryos come from for such research? There are only two sources: by collecting eggs from a woman's ovaries and fertilising them in vitro, or by flushing already fertilised eggs from her womb. Occasionally embryos are indeed flushed from their mothers, but it is an intrusive procedure and women are understandably reluctant to volunteer. Many more embryos are formed in vitro, for the purpose of helping the infertile. And of these there will always be some with three pronuclei, or that are cleaving badly, or are fragmented and distorted, so that they cannot be replaced in their mothers – they might grow abnormally or even threaten her life. Such embryos could be very valuable for research, however, and using them is little different from the long-established practice of using tissues from aborted fetuses.

Additionally, since it is usual as a back-up measure to fertilise more eggs than the three or four that will be replaced in a mother, there is often a surplus of perfectly normal embryos after a treatment has been completed. These spare embryos remain in vitro, awaiting their fate. Probably capable of growing into a baby, each can and should be frozen in case its mother needs it later. But when such frozen embryos are no longer needed by their parents, they must either be thrown away, donated to other couples, or used for research.

And finally, there are also special 'research embryos', created purely for experimental work. A woman coming to hospital for sterilisation or some other operation may agree to be given hormones so that her eggs may be collected and fertilised with donated sperm. These resulting embryos are then allocated for research.

Abnormal embryos, spare embryos, frozen embryos, research embryos – all these provide essential material for studies on early human life, studies of profound value to future men and women. But should these embryos be used? Should these studies be pursued?

# 5
# Ethical storms

These, then, are the main scientific procedures available to embryologists today, and just a few of the possibilities ahead. With so many technicalities involved there is clearly plenty of room for misunderstanding here — among scientists as well as non-scientists — and even when the precise facts are properly grasped there are still inevitably several highly controversial aspects. Furthermore, there are undeniably people and organisations whose gut-level opposition to the embryologist's work seems to lead them to jump with wilful eagerness to wrong and damaging conclusions.

In 1984, for example, I found myself the subject of a police investigation. A paper had been published describing my work, with other scientists, on the hormones released from embryos developing in a culture dish. The organisation LIFE, self-appointed to defend an extreme conservative moral stance, seized on one *en passant* detail in this paper, mentioning that an embryo had adhered to the plastic side of the dish, and claimed that the embryo had in fact 'implanted' (as if in a womb) in its culture vessel. It had therefore become conclusively human, and its subsequent use for research purposes constituted deliberate and grievous harm to a fellow human being.

The police were informed, and they did their duty. They called on me, made courteously detailed enquiries, and referred the matter to the Government. No charge was brought, for there was of course no case to answer. Apart from the fact that — rightly or wrongly — there is no law protecting such a very early embryo, LIFE was anyway completely mistaken in its basic assumption: the group of cells was *not* implanting, it was simply sticking to the plastic dish as any other disorganised group of cells might do.

LIFE's protest was a waste of everybody's time and money, and it could easily have been avoided if, instead of relying on their prejudices, they had taken the trouble to make a few quite elementary further enquiries.

Far more serious misunderstandings of my work had arisen in 1982. This was at a time when, as a result of intense public debate — ethical enquiries into IVF were being held by Protestant and Roman Catholic church authorities, by the Medical Research Council, the British Medical Association, the Royal College of Obstetricians and Gynaecologists, the Royal Society, and LIFE, to name just a few — the Government's Secretary of State for Social Services, Norman Fowler, had announced the setting-up of their own committee of enquiry, with a distinguished list of members headed by Mary Warnock.

Every conference organiser in Western Europe wanted ethics and embryos on his agenda and, among other places, I was asked to lecture at a medical journalists' gathering — to be held at Gatwick Airport, of all places. I accepted the invitation, but heard nothing more for several months and assumed that the idea had been abandoned. Then, suddenly and at very short notice, I was told that it was on after all. As I was by then committed on the day in question, being on duty in our Bourn Hall clinic, I agreed to telephone my lecture through for loudspeaker transmission in the conference hall just to help out the organisers. This is a somewhat unusual procedure at scientific meetings, but it was the best that could be done.

My lecture was pretty standard by then, and well-practised, and although there were clearly difficulties with the loudspeaker at the other end of the line while I was delivering it, everything seemed to go quite well. Next morning, however, my telephone started ringing. Reporters were asking for my response to comments in the day's papers. I hadn't yet read them, but when I did I was appalled.

Had the loudspeaker in the Gatwick conference hall really been so bad? The Press Association's report attacked embryo experiments I'd never performed, and a Dr Havard, Secretary to the BMA, was referring to cloning, which I didn't recommend, and implied that I was freezing embryos which I was not at the time. I attempted a denial, but it went virtually unheard. Dr Havard's attack was much more sensational: my ethical standards as a scientist were less stringent than those of doctors, he implied, and doctors should refuse to work with me except for accepted practices of fertilisation outside the body.

The headlines were dreadful.

'Test-tube mothers: call a halt.' (The *Standard*, 28 September, 1982)

'Don't work with this man.' (The *Daily Express*, 29 September, 1982)

This was too much to handle alone, so I called my solicitor. Apparently Dr Havard had tapes of the Gatwick meetings, so he was obviously pretty sure of himself. I must have said some awful things. We met Havard and I reluctantly issued a conciliatory statement with him, just to quieten the fuss. By now the journal *Hospital Doctor* had accused Patrick and me of being abortionists, and the BBC had for some reason revived the false accusation that we published only incomplete records of our work.

The following day, with a barrister now, I obtained copies of Dr Havard's tapes and we listened to them anxiously. First the lecture — that was clear enough and unequivocal: no grounds there for the many accusations. I breathed a sigh of relief. But there had been a question and answer session afterwards. Presumably I'd put my foot in it then.

We listened as the tape rolled on. One by one I answered

the questions in simple, straightforward terms, without misunderstandings on either side. I was innocent. Wherever my attackers had got their material it certainly wasn't from the Gatwick meeting!

'You've been grossly libelled,' my barrister told me. 'Havard's original statements are libels, and you could bring actions against every single newspaper that has repeated them . . . But I recommend that you concentrate on three — against the Press Association for an incorrect report, against the *Daily Express* for the malicious headlines, and against Dr Havard and the BMA.'

'What about Patrick?' I asked. 'Hasn't he been libelled too?'

'Certainly Mr Steptoe has been libelled. You could initiate joint actions against *Hospital Doctor* and the BBC also.'

That would make five. And if just one of them failed we could lose everything: money, reputation, all that we'd worked for down twenty years. But our reputations were in danger anyway, especially mine, and there had simply been too many insults. They had to be stopped.

'Issue all five,' I said.

Later that very same day my barrister and I were in touch again. *The Times* had published a surprisingly ill-judged editorial:

'By giving the impression that things are being done concealed from the public eye, and that embryos have been allowed to pass out of the protection of medical ethics, Dr Edwards does a disservice to the cause of research in his own field . . . He and other researchers would be wise to restrict themselves to procedures that directly serve the fertility treatments already generally accepted, and defer more controversial experiments until the present examination of these questions is complete and conclusions have been drawn.'

'That's another libel,' the barrister advised me.

'Start that action too,' I told him.

What difference would one more make? Six libel actions, against some of the most prestigious bodies in British society. What a prospect!

Encouragingly, *The Times* hastened to settle out of court, realising their mistake in uncritically accepting the Press Association's report. We decided to claim no damages, but it was very important that their apology should be printed in the leader column, where it would be sure to be noticed, exactly where the original libel had appeared.

The apology was fine: 'We accept that Dr Edwards has not done, nor has he suggested that he has done, anything concealed from the public eye, and we recognise that he and his colleagues have fully published the results of their work, and have repeatedly called for discussion of the ethical implications.' (*The Times*, 4 October 1982)

But unfortunately the apology appeared separated from the leader column by another item, so that its impact was seriously weakened, and I was advised that the matter must go to the High Court after all. The proceedings there were brief but impressive, and entirely in our favour.

*Hospital Doctor* decided to settle next then the Press Association. And so it went on. By 1984 even the BBC and the *Daily Express* were willing to settle and finally the BMA, ts settlement contributing further to our research funds. How the libels came about in the first place was never explained. But even today the issues raised remain bitterly contentious, and admittedly not without good reason.

One of the difficulties is that ethical controls are a systematised part of a doctor's daily life, as he makes decisions concerning abortions, contraceptive pills, or whether to tell a patient about his cancer, while scientists in general are left very much to find their own way.

A doctor's ethical position is laid down early in his career, with the Hippocratic oath: 'I swear by Apollo the healer . . . the regimen I adopt shall be for the benefit of the patients according to my ability and not for their hurt or any wrong . . .'

Furthermore this oath, sufficient in the past, is now regularly modified to keep up with developments in medical science: in attempting to define the difficult boundary between research and therapy, for example, the Helsinki Declaration states, 'Medical progress is based on research which ultimately must rest in part on experimentation involving human subjects . . .' New drugs give rise to new treatments requiring new research, so doctors live with batteries of regulations, and with a General Medical Council to establish guidelines, and hospital ethical committees, and colleges and associations.

'Any abuse by a doctor of any of the privileges and opportunities afforded to him, or any grave dereliction of professional duty, or serious breach of medical ethics, may give rise to a charge of serious professional misconduct . . .' (*Professional Conduct and Discipline: Fitness to Practise*, General Medical Council, 1981)

Doctors' organisations also stand ready for their defence in law, and their protection agencies are ready with advice, or to defend cases on their behalf.

Scientists, on the other hand, are very seldom taught ethics in their degree courses, their societies concentrate on research, and few of their laboratories have ethical committees. Animal licensing laws may curtail their freedom to do the sorts of experiment that most of them wouldn't want to do anyway, but in the main they don't look outside their laboratories for society's approval unless they happen to need funds. In that situation the criteria applied are all too often scientific rather than ethical.

So it is not surprising that 'What can be done will be done' is the charge often levelled at scientists. And it is not surprising that their critics demand commissions of enquiry as science ploughs relentlessly on, swamping the media with its successes, and awarding its most coveted prizes to those first past the post, making them stars overnight, as if the race and the winning were all that mattered.

For many non-scientists, who often see themselves as the only people truly in touch with reality, 'man the technician' has become a term of ultimate scorn. Most scientists simply ignore such attitudes, too busy with their own affairs. Not that it's entirely the scientists' fault their work turns sour in the public mind. Scientists, undeniably, designed and built the atom bomb, but it was non-scientists who ordered and paid for the redirection of nuclear research from peaceful to warlike ends. Scientists made the contraceptive pill, but it was the non-scientists' failure to provide strong moral leadership that resulted in teenage promiscuity and the spread of venereal diseases.

From where I stand, however, it's not all that significant that non-scientists are less than perfect. Scientists too have a lot to answer for. They need all the help they can get, and it was with this in mind, nearly twenty years ago, that a young American lawyer, Dave Sharpe, and I wrote a heartfelt piece in *Nature* magazine:

. . . perhaps what is needed is not heavy-handed public stature, or rule-making committees, or the conscience of individual doctors, but a simple organisation easily approached and consulted, to advise and assist biologists and others to reach their own decisions . . . It would frame public debate, act as a watchdog, and yet interfere minimally with the independence of science . . . Advisors are needed whose achievements and attitudes make them worth listening to in matters affecting the future of human research − doctors, scientists, lawyers, authors and other laymen − because they are broadly talented people.

Rulings should be as altruistic and detached as possible, powers of subpoena, funding research, or veto over particular work should be avoided as inconsistent with the advisory role . . . The stress would be on individual and private action, enquiry and consultation, not on authority, bureaucracy, or 'laws with teeth' . . .

When scientists clearly foresee potential conflicts with existing rules of society arising from their work, paradoxically both human progress and scientific freedom may hang on their activism in arenas generally regarded as social or political. Scientists may have to make disclosures of their work and its consequences that run against their immediate interests; they may have to stir up public opinion, even lobby for laws before legislatures, in the hope that the attitudes of society as evidenced in its laws will mature at a rate not too far behind the transition of scientific discovery into technological achievement. The lob-byists for reform in the laws of drug and alcohol abuse, abortion and sexual behaviour have achieved much public approval in their areas of concern; can biologists in experimental embry-ology expect so much more by doing any less?' (Edwards and Sharpe, *Nature* 231 (1971), 87–91)

At the time there was hardly any response. The British Association for the Advancement of Science put together a panel of politicians, theologians, doctors and scientists to consider IVF and related matters, and later produced a book on the subject (*Our Future Inheritance, Choice or Chance*, W.F. Bodmer and A. Jones, Oxford University Press, 1974) but it was completely overlooked. It took the birth of Louise Brown to arouse serious public interest, but by then the field was one in which many of the important decisions had already been taken in Oldham, by ourselves and the local ethical committee.

And others were taken soon afterwards. At the British Medical Research Council, for instance, their doctors and scientists had started and continued working with research embryos. The increasing public pressure in the early 1980s obliged the Council to hold an enquiry and issue the official directive that such research was acceptable – but only to the 'implantation stage', whatever that might mean. Still, at least their staff could now work in peace, content that what they had long been doing anyway was now officially legitimate. We ourselves had been working with spare or abnormal embryos, but as our freezing programme was introduced, we decided that the spare embryos should be frozen instead for later replacement into their mothers, so we were left only with the abnormal embryos.

During these years, and ever since, I have written and spoken about ethics on every conceivable occasion. In the early years of IVF, though, we alone could not inform the whole of society properly on the facts of the matter. Otherwise, this serious failure would have left the field open to our most emotional opponents, many of whom are skilful manipulators of public opinion at the expense of public knowledge.

Cloning in particular, as I've already said, has come to typify everything suspicious about embryo research, with pictures conjured up by the ignorant of whole football teams of identical, all-conquering players, and of millionaires paying out fortunes for a perverted sort of immortality. Horror stories in books and plays describe how an Einstein or a Hitler is copied a hundred times and more, to relive their lives in nightmare, zombie-like repetition. At one intellectual level, philosophers thoughtfully debate the value to society of clones of specially talented people, and at another level the popular German journal *Stern* titillates its readers with tales of demented armies of rapists and murderers.

The fact is, it cannot be done at present and, on the scale imagined, it probably never will be. And even if it could be, the resulting clones would not grow up to reproduce their single parent slavishly: environment plays an immeasurably important part in human development, and neither good nor evil genius will survive differences in generation, society and place. Identical twins separated at birth might discover they are alike in some astonishing ways when they meet again as adults, but they will have grown very differently in many others. And even if good or evil genius *does* survive across generations, the whole operation seems to me such an improbable waste of time and money. No individual could justify being cloned until he or she had been proved as an adult, so that clones must necessarily be at least twenty-five years younger than their parent. And who can possibly predict the genetic needs of the next generation? We call it 'clowning'.

Obviously a lot of the cloning talk is only meant as fun. But it rubs off on the science it clumsily borrows. Somewhere, often unrecognised at the backs of people's minds, the picture lingers of the embryologist as a mad scientist, busily cloning monsters. And not all the people who think like that are fools. Even a doctor as distinguished as Professor Ian Donald, the pioneer of ultrasound and the first man to give me human eggs for ripening in vitro, has been reported in the *Daily Telegraph* as fearing hybrid experiments, the creation of human beings from embryo to childbirth outside the womb, and the cloning of 'Hitlerite hordes' of identical babies unless a stop is put to experimentation now.

For many people these are undeniably genuine fears – of ectogenesis, animal uterine hosts, man/animal hybrids – and nature does indeed permit some unusual permutations. Horses can gestate zebras, species hybrids do exist, and chimaeras have been known to survive – an animal, for example, that is composed half of goat and half of sheep cells. Such phenomena teach scientists more and more about life and its mysteries, but only an unbalanced doctor or scientist would want to attempt such techniques upon humankind, and insanity, with its attendant dangers, is a risk that exists in any profession.

As to the 'only meant as fun' argument, it can be dangerous. Back in 1986 rumours got about concerning the establishment of pregnancy in men: Oxford studies on cancer before had shown that mouse blastocysts could implant in a testis, and human fetuses are well known to grow occasionally on the ovary or in the abdomen of a woman, so it was suggested that the same could be done in men, by implanting embryos in an intestine.

An article in *Newsweek* for 14 July that year was headlined: 'The New Motherhood . . . The French news weekly, *Le Nouvel Observateur*, recently found that one in three Frenchmen under thirty-five would . . . consider bearing a child. Suddenly male pregnancy is one of the hot topics in Europe.'

Even though such ectopic pregnancies are dangerous and life-threatening, unacceptable under any circumstances, a scientific joke had suddenly become serious business, with queues of men reportedly waiting for the treatment. And once again, foolish though they may be, such follies rub off on the medical profession. Embryologists are seen as irresponsible at best, criminally insane at worst.

Not meant as fun at all was yet another claim, also in 1986, that scientists in America had separated male and female spermatozoa and that patients would therefore be able to choose the sex of their children.

'Doctors yesterday announced the birth to a New Orleans couple of what they said was the first test-tube baby whose sex had been predetermined,' ran a story in the *Guardian* that August.

Fears were voiced of a nationwide change in the ratio of the sexes if choice became possible. But the technique was in fact an old one, whereby early inseminations are believed to produce a girl and later inseminations a boy, and it has long been proved false. Even so, endless similar claims continue to surface.

'Are we wise enough to be allowed to select a baby's gender?' the *Washington Post* asked, commenting on an over-the-counter kit that was being marketed, promising to predetermine a baby's sex. They needn't have worried, for on investigation this turned out to be an old and disproved method too. Now, however, the Japanese have climbed on the sexing bandwagon, with a slight change in technique that claims to give a boy or girl virtually at will – and the procedure has reportedly been banned by the Japanese government. Whether or not this new method will turn out to be as unsound as its predecessors (in December 1988) remains to be seen.

Nevertheless, in today's media-oriented world it is inevitably the flashy claims – no matter how unfounded – that become front-page news, while the sober rebuttals lie unnoticed somewhere at the bottom of page three. So it is the follies that linger in the public mind. Thus man the

technician is seen as blinkered and inhumane. This preference of the headline writers for the sensational is hard to
fight — the actual facts will often be both dull and difficult to
understand. Scientists have a duty, however, to make sure
that they *are* understood: it is a duty we have too long been
shirking.

'Suddenly, technology and science seem to have out-
stripped existing ethics,' wrote Margaret Jay in a December
1981 issue of the *Listener*.

If she meant that 'suddenly' in all seriousness, one could
only wonder where Ms Jay had been during all the scientific
dramas of the previous decade. Still, her comment was
basically true — and anyway, perhaps she's right, and in the
measured progress of ethical systems, developments over
ten or fifteen years may indeed be termed sudden.

Certainly, as we shall see in following chapters, the
responses of many of the traditional ethical arbiters to the
new situations created by scientific advance seem hasty and
misinformed, almost bordering on a panic reaction.

# 6
# The argument

The basic question involved in the ethics of embryo research and in-vitro fertilisation has to centre on the status of the human embryo, its rights and the duties we owe it, and consequently whether it should be conceived in vitro for research, only for IVF or other therapies, or not at all.

The status of the human embryo appears a simple matter. It is alive, and it is neither a hamster nor a chicken — it is human. And an undeniable law of creation would seem to be that every species looks after its own. Nevertheless, the status of the human embryo is a question that taxes to the full the minds of theologians and philosophers, as well as the more practical men and women of law and politics. It taxes the minds of scientists too, whether Christian or Humanist, Jew, Muslim or Hindu. And at present, frankly, the only outcome of all this thought is a well-meaning but ultimately dangerous confusion.

Western societies in general rate early embryonic life fairly low. They sanction intra-uterine devices or morning-after pills, both of which expel embryos aged five days or more from the mother's womb, and they increasingly accept 'interceptives' or 'contragestives' which remove life support from fetuses of fourteen days and even older. They permit abortion too, often for no other reason than that the fetus is inconvenient, the outcome of a failed contraceptive. Malformed fetuses are aborted also, if the parents feel they cannot cope, or if the degree of malformation is considered too severe to allow a decent quality of life were the child to come to full term. Such decisions are painful, and humanely intentioned, but it has to be said that they are dangerously subjective. And furthermore, societies then permit the tissues of these abortuses to be used for research purposes, to produce vaccines, to study organ growth, or for therapeutic grafting into recipients.

'A consistent and informed [expression] of the respect due to human life,' the *Economist* pointed out in 1986, '. . . is precisely what countries do not have if they agonise over embryo research and yet condone abortion.'

Confusion indeed.

'We are being brought to the brink of something almost like the atom bomb. The potential of what can be done is quite horrific,' said Sir John Peel, a one-time President of the Royal College of Obstetricians and Gynaecologists, of embryo research. Yet he chaired a commission that came out with the Peel Report in 1972: 'The use of the whole pre-viable fetus is permissible provided that . . . the minimal limit of viability should be regarded as twenty weeks gestational age . . .' And this is the report that still governs research upon the tissues of abortuses in Britain – and most other western societies follow similar guidelines. A government commission has now been established to review this report.

It is hardly surprising that all the fuss about studying fertilised eggs and embryos only a few days old seems needlessly theatrical to many people, when they realise what may be done to well-formed fetuses at five months gestation.

Has the battle for embryos' rights already been lost, then? Is it open season on these minute early stages of human life, a day or two after fertilisation, these blastocysts far too small to be seen by the naked eye? Certainly not. Embryos have property rights, if few others. In law they can inherit their father's estate if he dies while they are in their mother's womb, provided simply that they survive to be born alive. They can also claim damages in most countries for injury inflicted in the womb, provided again that they are born alive, but with the added requirement in Britain that they survive a further forty-eight hours.

More confusion. Embryos have retrospective rights to property, and to court-awarded damages, and not to life itself. Clearly an embryo's rights before the law are no shining example of incisive legal thinking.

But Britain claims to be a Christian country, and certainly the Christian churches have a powerful voice in our government's decisions, so what about an embryo's rights before God? And here, from the Roman Catholic Church, we are given what appears to be a wholly consistent and unequivocal opinion.

The Roman Catholic Church has judged matters of reproduction for centuries, has been wrong before, and has admitted it — for instance, the medieval Church's now modified belief in baptism as the only alternative to hellfire for even the tiniest dying fetuses. This led to all thirty-seven 'babies' being solemnly baptized after being delivered at one birth in the year 1269 by the unfortunate Countess Margaret of Cracow (we suspect now that her pregnancy must have been a hydatidiform mole, a grossly swollen placenta brought about when an embryo grows only with its father's chromosomes, the many watery vesicles of which were mistaken for fetuses).

The Roman Catholic Church is also misinformed over matters of reproduction and sex today — for instance, it describes homosexuality as 'unnatural' (a curious word to use for only one particular aspect of a species that has come as far from its natural world of the forest as *homo sapiens*) and therefore a sin, even though homosexuality is now believed often to be chromosomal, a matter of genetic inheritance, or a psychological consequence of upbringing.

Possibly none of this matters. Churchmen, like everyone else, do the best they can with the information at their disposal, and firm guidance is useful, if only as an arguing point.

The official Roman Catholic position is clear, and

absolutist. The moment of fertilisation establishes a human being, and therefore — as with all forms of abortion — all research on human embryos is fundamentally unacceptable. Freezing should be outlawed also, and IVF, and embryo selection. Such absolutism was made official in 1987 by the Vatican's Congregation for the Doctrine of the Faith: in-vitro fertilisation contravened an embryo's right to be conceived in marriage, freezing offended the dignity due to human beings, donation broke the genetic continuity of the family, research was illicit unless the embryos suffered no harm, and pre-natal diagnosis should be restricted to purely therapeutic procedures on a fetus.

'It is immoral to produce human embryos destined to be exploited as "biological material" . . . Depriving them at least temporarily of material shelter and gestation [by freezing them] is placing them in a situation in which further offences and manipulations are possible.

'. . . Marriage does not confer on spouses the right to have a child, but only the right to perform those natural acts which are *per se* ordered to procreation.'

Required to support the Bible's injunction to be fruitful and multiply, Roman Catholic bishops may claim to welcome scientific advances that enable infertile couples to have children, but it is a very limited welcome. For these are the bishops who declared, in their 1983 Joint Committee on Bioethical Issues, that test-tube babies were in some way less than human because they could not claim their 'origin in a single act, an act of love or friendship or mutual involvement and commitment, and an act equally of my parents and of them alone . . .'

In a book published a year earlier, in 1982, the Roman Catholic Archbishop of Melbourne, Monsignor Frank Little, asked a moral question of those practising in-vitro fertilisation:

'One must first ask whether Professor Wood and those associated with him had the moral right to embark on a procedure which placed them in the predicament of "destruction or freezing" . . . Should we not commence with the fundamental principle: God has bound the transmission of human life to the conjugal sex act . . . If science seeks to exclude or substitute for the marital act, the scientific action is not licit.'

His question deserves a straight scientific answer. It was clinical urgency that gave the doctors the moral right, the necessity even, to embark on the procedure. The archbishop should be told also that it was evolution, rather than an arbitrary, one-off act of God, that bound the transmission of life to the sex act, and that the connection is therefore always open to modification or abandonment.

Archbishop Hume, however, the senior Roman Catholic in Britain, is firmly on Archbishop Little's side – so much so that he withdrew his patronage from the Royal Society for Mentally Handicapped Children and Adults when that society decided to approve embryo research within the limits laid down in the Warnock Report. Here is an extract from a radio interview he gave on the BBC's *World at One* news programme on 23 January 1986:

*Interviewer:* But MENCAP is only endorsing research on embryos in an attempt to prevent handicaps in future generations of children. How can you really say that's wrong?

*Hume:* Because the Catholic position is perfectly clear – that from the actual moment of conception human life is there, and I don't make the distinction between pre-embryo and embryo. It is human life: it is a continuum from the moment of conception to where we find ourselves today. If we agree that it is not right to experiment on and then destroy embryos, then you may not experiment on one embryo for the good of another. The whole idea of freezing embryos, the whole idea of selling and buying embryos which this policy would entail is – humanly speaking – difficult to accept.

*Interviewer:* So you'd say, really it was better to accept the suffering that handicap involves, than to conduct this sort of experimentation?

*Hume:* Yes, I do. Because I really believe firmly that there is a
pattern to life, which is God's pattern, and which is often
difficult for us to understand. I realise, of course, this pre-
supposes a belief in God and in His love for us, and that
things may sometimes work out differently from what
we expect. We should not confine ourselves to a vision
of life, and of this world, which does not go beyond this
present life.

There are Roman Catholic theologians who go still
further. In his book *Begotten or Made?* (Clarendon Press,
Oxford, 1984) Oliver O'Donovan seems to fear progress
itself. Why do we want a better world? he asks. Technology
mechanises life, he claims, so that nothing is 'natural' any
more: mass media control politics, analytical methods
regulate love, and children are begotten by surgical
intervention. Instead, he suggests, Christians should con-
fess their faith in God's natural order as declared in the Old
Testament, they should 'act well' and believe in human
brotherhood.

He has a point. In Old Testament days responsibility and
family feeling (the brotherhood of man) were passed on
fruitfully in levirate marriages, when a widow married her
dead husband's brother as a matter of course. But today the
world is rather more complicated. Women are no longer
men's chattels, for one thing.

Writing in the 1984 *Journal of Medical Ethics*, another
Roman Catholic thinker, Teresa Iglesias, adds her support.
Human embryos from the very outset are sacrosanct,
untouchable, unownable, characterised by structure and
organisation, persons in their own right. Uncontrolled
science, she says (as if such a thing were ever suggested), will
transform *Homo sapiens* into *Homo mechanicus*.

At least, by maintaining ruthless consistency, the Roman
Catholic Church seems to be keeping things simple for its
followers. But it is an illusory simplicity, as I have already
shown, since it depends upon a single moment of fertilisation linked to a single creation of human potential, while in

reality the potential is not finalised even at birth. And in fact there is conflict among even the most conservative elements of the Church, as problems of ensoulment are argued — in other words, the exact moment when the soul enters the human embryo — especially since they now know that several days after fertilisation must elapse before anyone can be certain that a particular embryo is not so seriously malformed as to be incapable of independent life, or monstrous, significantly other than human.

'It seems extraordinary,' writes one distinguished philosopher, Jean M. Mill, in the 1986 *Journal of Medical Ethics*, 'that some people propose . . . microbiological techniques ought to be applied in twentieth-century medicine by a consideration of how . . . Aristotle's . . . categories of thought apply to the concept of being . . . Until the embryo becomes dependent upon, or is related to, the person, I can see no reason for regarding it as human or personal. It seems to me correct to call it biological.'

Furthermore, one step down from the Church's rulers there is serious disunity.

A Roman Catholic theologian, John Mahoney, has written a closely-reasoned book on the subject of bioethics (*Bioethics and Belief*, Sheed & Ward, London, 1984). He questions the motives of scientists, wonders how they relate to society, to culture, to religious beliefs, and is worried about the value of knowledge that is gained by dubious methods. But he is sympathetic towards in-vitro fertilisation if practised between husband and wife, and therefore towards masturbation for that same purpose. He accepts frozen embryos, even research embryos, and also contraception.

Much of this he derives from a very detailed reassessment of the embryo's status: 'to describe the conceptus as only potentially a human person is to ignore the fact that even the child at birth is still only potentially a human person . . . Those who claim this description of a potential human person applies exclusively to the embryo or foetus at an early stage are using the term "potential" to mean that it is not yet in any real sense a person at all.

'[Arguments about natural law] frequently spring from a mentality which prefers to canonise the past and the familiar than to explore the unknown and the future . . . . In this it is profoundly mistaken . . . the difference is one between the passive acceptance of God's gifts, and finding in them the challenge of active stewardship.'

Mahoney discusses problems of ensoulment, embryos that die soon after fertilisation, genetically abnormal foetuses, identical twins, and the significance of brain development — in particular the appearance of the neo-cortex (the feature that many people would claim makes us uniquely human) at some time between the twenty-fifth and the fortieth day.

Sadly, he had to pay a price for his open-mindedness. His book examined too many controversial questions, and Archbishop Hume publicly withdrew his imprimatur in July 1986.

Another questioning Roman Catholic, this time in America, suffered an even worse fate as a result of his stance on the moral issues of sexuality and reproduction in the modern world. The Vatican stripped Charles Curran of his right to teach theology at the Roman Catholic University in Washington: the Archbishop of Washington, Chancellor of the University, announced that he was not 'suitable or eligible to teach Catholic theology'. And then, despite Curran's endorsement by his own American Catholic Theological Society, the Vatican reached out a few weeks later to ban him from teaching altogether.

Although he has since taken successful legal action against the right of the Vatican to prevent him teaching in an American university, he is at present understandably reluctant to take advantage of the judgment by resuming his work against the Vatican's wishes.

Clearly, as *The Times* correspondent C. Longley put it on 4 August 1986, the Vatican's Sacred Congregation for the

Doctrine of the Faith has decided 'to enforce by discipline a consensus in the Church on sexual morality which does not really exist.'

And what had Curran done? He had written articles which accepted the break between sex and procreation if a greater value were served. He had welcomed in-vitro ferilisation when it involved husband and wife, had suggested that an embryo's status might change in the days following fertilisation, and had seen the possibility that the rights of individuals might have to be balanced against the beneficial consequences of certain actions.

'Through technology and science man has been able to improve his lot in this world,' he wrote. 'There is a definite possibility that in the future, and to some extent even now, man can eliminate deleterious genes from the human gene pool, which will improve human individuals and the human species . . . From the outset of these discussions, we must realise that the relationship between the scientist and ethician is not one of opposition or exclusion.

'The Christian vision of man and his world cannot accept any Utopian schemes. Modern life and science do give man much greater dominion than he had before, but man remains a creature and a sinner. The final stage of the reign of God is in the future and not totally continuous with man's present existence.'

A sane attitude promising fruitful discussion, one might have thought, and certainly an attitude supported not only by American Catholics but also by the British Catholic Theological Association and many others. Even so, although it was sane, it was neither simple nor unequivocal. And so Curran had to go. The Vatican also stripped the Archbishop of Seattle, Raymond Hundhausen, of his authority in several pastoral areas, for expressing similarly liberal views.

On 12 November 1986, a *Times* correspondent reported from America: 'American Roman Catholic bishops have been meeting in Washington this week in an atmosphere of crisis, as recent Vatican actions against liberal Catholics and pronouncements on sexual morality have stirred up widespread anger here and threaten to cause a schism within the US Catholic Church.'

Threatened schisms, as seen by reporters, are usually serious overstatements. But in the same day's *Independent* the President of the US National Conference of Catholic Bishops, Bishop James Malone, was reported as saying that the Pope's insistence on doctrinal orthodoxy was leading to 'a growing and dangerous disaffection of elements of the Church in the United States from the Holy See'.

It was a time when lay US Roman Catholics, too, some having been treated by in-vitro fertilisation, rejected the Doctrine of the Faith.

One went on record: 'God and I are just fine.'

Another, a woman currently going through an in-vitro fertilisation procedure with her husband, said, 'I am very disappointed in my church . . . They have just lost a couple of Catholics.'

Obviously a church, even more than any other organisation, has to provide moral leadership rather than simply be swayed by a few very vocal protestors. But leadership that is excessively doctrinaire may well lose credibility and become worse than no leadership at all. And possibly the Vatican was recognising this, for compromise followed.

In October 1986, *The Times* reported: 'Catholics may use the pill after rape.' The recommendation had come from the Joint Committee on Bioethical Issues, one of the Church's more conservative agencies: morning-after pills were now allowed, pills which expelled fertilised embryos from the womb. Less than consistent, no doubt, since such contraception was still forbidden to married or consenting couples — which suggested that an embryo resulting from rape was somehow less human than one more gently conceived — but a humane step and surely a conciliatory one.

And in a 1987 pamphlet published by the Catholic Truth Society, *Catholics and AIDS, Questions and Answers*, the use of condoms is recommended as a preventative measure. A Vatican archbishop, Fiorenzo Angelini, would not endorse this recommendation — 'It is not realistic to talk about these devices,' he is reported as saying in January 1988 — but in fact the compromise offered by this recommendation seems extremely realistic. It has a respectable provenance too, expressing the Church's long-held doctrine of the Double Effect, which forgives a minor sin if committed to avoid a greater.

To summarise: the Roman Catholic Church's stand on the rights and status of the embryo is not as unequivocal as it appears at first sight. Pope Paul I was reported to have been delighted for the first test-tube mother. There are church members also, like the philosopher Bernard Häring, who suggest that the development of the neo-cortex might be the decisive indication of human potential, which would move the embryo's personhood on to somewhere between the twenty-fifth and the fortieth day . . . I do not wish to imply here that such uncertainties are a bad thing, or a sign of weakness. These are complex issues, and simple, narrow answers will never be sufficient. Any opening-out of the debate has to be healthy.

Anglican churchmen, although perhaps historically less doctrinaire, are similarly confused. Back in 1948 the then Archbishop of Canterbury condemned donor insemination as an immoral act. Today semen and egg donation still worry the bishops' synod, as does surrogacy, since it sees these measures for some not very clear reason as threats to the traditional Christian marriage. And the present Archbishop of Canterbury, a far more open-minded church leader than many, is clearly regretting some aspects of his own long-standing liberalism: 'I used to be rather glib,' he is reported as saying, in *The Times* for 30 March 1987, 'about this idea that with greater knowledge, moral horizons are enlarged. But I have become uncomfortable with these arguments . . . [much] of our shallow morality springs from this lack of a sense of wonder. My . . . moral attitudes should fit not into the logic of thinking which could be the same for a humanist or a believer, but fit adequately into my vision of God's love for us . . .'

One difficulty has to be that recently the Anglican Church's authority — particularly in scientific or sexual matters — has become seriously blurred. From within its own ranks fundamental tenets such as the Virgin Birth and the Resurrection have come under fire. Also, although the Church of England has temporised in its handling of its homosexual clergy, thus responding at least tentatively to new scientific knowledge and society's changing views, it has still been willing to persevere in refusing women the right to ordination. Even if this particular attitude seems to be changing, with its American branch having installed Rev. Barbara Harris as Bishop of Massachusetts (*The Times*, 2 August 1988), these failures of leadership seem all the more distressing since there is, in general, a questioning spirit alive in its members.

As the Anglican Board of Social Responsibility wrote in 1985: 'The creative process continues and involves ever-widening horizons of human knowledge and capability. We are in the midst of a journey whose beginnings lay in creation and whose end is to be realised in the hope given to us in Jesus Christ.'

On the subject of embryo research in particular, the distinguished Anglican, Clifford Longley, has written: 'There appears to be no act of faith by means of which a conviction can be gained that [human] life begins at fertilisation.' While an American colleague, John Fletcher, who works at first hand with severely handicapped children and their parents, bravely tries to answer the age-old apparent nonsense of a supposedly loving Christian God who nevertheless tolerates crippling genetic disasters such as spina bifida and Tay-Sachs disease: 'God is not indictable for events that involve evil, because evil is the result of decisions and outcomes for which God cannot be considered responsible, given a measure of self-determination on the part of each creature.' Sadly, he doesn't explain who actually is responsible for evil or for that unfortunate self-determination if God isn't. And another liberal thinker, Joseph Fletcher, has a sharp answer for those Roman Catholics who suggest that a test-tube baby must in some sense be less than human: 'A baby made artificially,' he writes, 'by deliberate and careful contrivance, would be more human than one resulting from sexual roulette . . . [which is] the reproductive mode of the human species.'

It hardly needs saying that, in historical terms, both Protestant and Roman Catholic churches have been slow to accept new scientific truths — from Galileo, through Darwin to Malthus and the contraception pioneers of the nineteenth and twentieth centuries, scientific innovators have seldom been given an easy time. But resistance to change — for the breathing space it gives, the opportunity for all concerned to check themselves and seriously consider — is not always a bad thing. Only when it is blind, and stultifies thought, is resistance damaging in the long term.

Most Christians recognise this, of course, and few more so than Lord Soper, leader of the British Methodists. In a 1984 debate on in-vitro fertilisation in the House of Lords, stating his faith and ethical position, he came outspokenly to terms with many recent scientific developments. His present world, he conceded, was significantly different from that which had helped him fashion his moral principles, in that many actions previously ascribed to God's omnipotent power alone now lay within man's competence. Furthermore, in making ethical judgments the Bible was only of limited assistance, as in its harsh judgments about homosexuality.

'I have to find my morality, at least in specific terms, in the processes of the Christian Church . . . [Yet it] very largely lays down its principles with regard to sexual morality in terms which [are] now completely out of date and quite wrong.'

Christian tradition, which taught that man was given the

active seed of life, to be implanted and imbedded in passive woman, had led to an exploitative, male-dominated society, and must be rejected. Compassion and the preservation of the family were fundamental Christian bases for ethical judgments, no morality was absolute, and the acceptance of compromises was anyway by no means new: the doctrine of a righteous war, for example, allowed those preaching the sanctity of human life to tolerate its indiscriminate destruction.

Lord Soper pointed out linguistic traps, too. 'We do not use words like "baby", "child", and "living creature" with great clarity: after all, a flower is alive, and so is a beetle . . .'

As a Christian minister he saw no reason to believe that the status of early embryos was equal to that of adult humans; donor insemination should be approached with compassion, since it worked towards the preservation of the family; and research on spare embryos was acceptable, since to allow them to die was no more moral than to make use of them in helping others, in easing others' suffering. And finally, he believed that the instruments of science gave him an opportunity to aspire to a more spiritual life, and for that he was grateful.

The Christian writer C.S. Lewis, on the other hand, laid down a basic theological abhorrence of all things scientific as long ago as 1943, in his document *The Abolition of Man*, and there is a school of churchmen that follows his teachings even now. These are readily identified by a number of emotive key words: dehumanisation, debiologisation, scientism, depersonalisation. Lewis' fears of science led him to see man's conquest of nature as similar to the tyranny of one nation over another, or of one generation of men over another.

This is the starting point for what is sometimes called the 'slippery slope' theory, through which its supporters consider a realistic view of man's base nature leads them to believe that every new discovery is bound to lead eventually to undesirable ends. While fashionably cynical, this theory is not wholly borne out by experience: some ends – atom bombs, for example – have certainly been undesirable, but many others, such as antibiotics or pain-free dentistry, would be harder to fault.

And besides, as the American biologist Clifford Grob-stein points out, 'All slopes, after all, do not end in precipices . . . We do not invariably forgo something that is basically beneficial because it may be abused or may lead toward something malignant. Rather we move to establish sound guidelines and policies that set appropriate boundaries . . .'

Clearly, then, there is little unanimity in the Christian churches on the status of the human embryo, or on the future of embryo research – every opinion exists, in fact, from wholesale prohibition to wholesale acceptance, with every possible shade of compromise in between. But these are vitally important questions, questions that ultimately we have to decide for ourselves, and we need all the help we can get, so what of the non-Christian philosophers? What advice do they give?

The humanists are unequivocal. In June 1988, the British Humanist Association announced: 'Conduct should be based on reason, evidence, understanding and toler-ance . . . We can see no convincing moral argument to stand in the way of embryo research.'

It has to be admitted, however, that since such philoso-phers operate rationally, like scientists, they have only limited popular appeal, for they have nothing of the numinous, nothing to match Christianity's sense of mys-tery, its ceremonies rich in dignity and pomp, its authority that is greater than human. But at least they stand, more successfully than most, outside political systems, eco-nomics, and socially conditioned emotions.

Some of their observations are startling, yet so obvious that one wonders why one hasn't seen them for oneself. The Australian philosopher, Helge Kuhse, points out, modifying Hume's famous dictum, that if scientists may be accused of playing God when they start life deliberately, then they also play God when they *don't* start it. For her, 'immoral' simply means 'contrary to the current standards of society', and she finds theology unhelpful: 'Theological ethics has only a limited appeal. But philosophical ethics, in contrast to faith-based ethics, addresses a universal audience, not a particular sub-group.'

Another philosopher, Harris, refuting the belief that an embryo's human potential automatically confers human status upon it, points out by analogy that although everyone will eventually die, it is hardly reasonable to treat them as if they were dead already.

Most philosophers are gradualists. They believe that an embryo grows from 'organism' to 'being' to 'person' as it passes from fertilisation, through birth to childhood. To them the question 'when does embryonic life begin?' is less important than the question, 'when does embryonic life begin to matter morally?'

Lockwood sets great store by brain development: 'I identify far more strongly with the laboratory rabbit that, like me, sees, feels and suffers, and has a brain, than with a primitive, insensate, and literally brainless clump of cells.'

While discussing human potential, he also questions the value of moral decisions based on identical twins, since 'split-brained' adults have two streams of consciousness. He worries if knowledge of embryology is itself enough to draw moral conclusions. Anyway, if nature itself chooses to defer definitive identity until well into the gestation period, who are we to differ?

Indeed, for some philosophers it is not until the moment of full self-consciousness that a child becomes truly human, a viewpoint that hardly helps the debate about embryos! Others such as the Australian Peter Singer question the basic anthropocentricity of the debate, suggesting that each individual monkey, rat or sparrow is as genetically unique as any human, and should be treated as such. Recent claims that chimpanzees have been taught standard deaf persons' sign language lend support to the proposition that we humans are less 'special' than we like to believe. If that should be the case, then the whole debate is given an entirely new dimension.

Mary Warnock's philosophy — of particular interest because of the influential committee she headed — leads her to withold human status from the embryo until it has become a full human being, but she carefully avoids a direct answer as to when exactly that moment occurs. Instead, like the law lord, Lord Devlin, she prefers popular emotion as the final arbiter, agreeing with Hume that mortality is 'more properly felt than judged of'.

In the foreword to her committee's report she writes: 'Moral questions . . . involve not only a calculation of the consequences, but also strong sentiments with regard to the nature of the proposed activities . . .'

Many philosophers find this a dubious proposal. Harris, for one, points out that 'Not all feelings, however strongly held, are moral feelings'. Lord Devlin, when he argued similarly during a debate on homosexuality some years ago that morals should be judged by reasonable rather than rational men, was widely ridiculed. According to him, his critics said, an act is immoral 'if the thought of it makes the man on the Clapham omnibus sick'.

Harris castigates feelings on their own still further when he comments on the use of pictures of fetuses to make moral points. 'Why should we not assume that the empathy evoked by the sight of a three-month-old fetus is just a soggy sentimentality, classically evoked by . . . creatures like puppies?'

The French philosopher, Jacques Monod, goes even deeper, criticising the basic animism that sees man as a perfect product of the past, an ordered being. 'Modern societies accept the treasures and the power offered them by science. But they have not accepted . . . its profounder message: the defining of a new and unique source of truth, and the demand for a thorough revision of ethical premises, for a complete break with the animist tradition . . . Enjoying all the riches they owe to science, our societies are still trying to live by and to teach systems of values already blasted at the root by science itself.'

And finally, after the philosophers have had their say, the women's liberation movement contributes its own perspective. Feminists in general place little emphasis on defining the status of the human embryo. Prompted perhaps by an intense sympathy for their fellow women and angered by the cradle mentality a predominantly male society forces upon them, they concentrate on ends rather than means: in short, the self-determination that embryo research can bring them. Women, they argue, are the individuals most closely concerned when any decision is taken concerning reproductive processes. They ask principally for information and consultation. In any conflict between the interests of embryo and mother, they have no doubt whose should prevail. And for the rest, many are pragmatic, seeing the eventual benefits of research as paramount. If Mary Warnock is right, such priorities will count heavily in philosophical decision-making.

Inevitably I have put together here no more than a very brief and imperfect summary of the embryology debate. Every day, as new possibilities open up, new arguments for and against will be advanced. This chapter is meant simply to be a starting point, and a few clues to the shape of the terrain and its pitfalls. But the argument itself is one that we must all join in, for only then can we take a useful part in the decisions that have to be made. Otherwise we leave these decisions to others – to the politicians or the lawyers – and this is a serious failure. In such vital matters democracy can only function properly with our active participation.

# 7
# The Warnock Committee

In July 1982, in response to intense public concern, the British government established a committee of inquiry into human fertilisation and embryology, under the chairmanship of Dame, now Lady Mary Warnock, Mistress of Girton College, Cambridge, for the purpose of examining 'the social, ethical, and legal implications of recent and potential developments in the field of human assisted reproduction'. By thus taking official notice of the embryology controversy the British government led the world, but was soon followed by other governments in Europe and Australia. In the USA, however, although the matter is of at least equal importance there, the division of power between the states and the federal government has so far prevented any official attempt at a similar, nationwide consensus.

The Warnock Committee, as it immediately came to be known, was comprised of sixteen members, five women and eleven men, and included distinguished theologians, a director of the Dartington North Devon Trust, two social workers, three men trained in the law, eight members of the medical and scientific professions, and the philosopher, Dame Mary Warnock, herself. They had two joint secretaries and a legal adviser, and two senior civil servants were present as observers.

The committee sat for nearly two years. Its brief was very broad, it heard an enormous amount of evidence, and its final report amounted to some ninety-three pages, which include several dissenting opinions. It makes interesting reading, if only as a comment upon the attitudes and opinions of sixteen intelligent, concerned and well-informed British citizens in the first half of the 1980s.

As an indication of the thoroughness of the report's approach I shall quote first from its introductory chapter and then, because the subsequent parliamentary debate considered them as a whole and because selecting from them would be an impertinence anyway, I shall give its recommendations in full.

Chapter One.
Scope of the Inquiry.

In considering our terms of reference, we recognised that we were being asked to examine a sphere of activity still developing, and rapidly changing. A common factor linking all the developments, recent or potential, medical or scientific, was the anxiety which they generated in the public mind. We have therefore looked at the new processes of assisted reproduction, including surrogacy, which can cause public concern. We have also considered artificial insemination which, although practised in this country for many years, is not universally accepted ethically, nor indeed regulated by law. There were, however, some matters which, although in some sense related, fell outside our terms of reference. Chief among these were contraception and abortion. We have not concerned ourselves directly with these, although the present state of the law in relation to them has been a necessary point of reference in discussions . . .

Methods of working.

We found it convenient to divide our task into two parts. The first concerned processes designed to benefit the individual within society who faced a particular problem, namely infertility; the second concerned the pursuit of knowledge, much of it designed to benefit society at large rather than the individual . . .

Role of the Inquiry.

We have confined our recommendations to certain practical proposals, capable of implementation. We have tried to frame these recommendations in general terms, leaving matters of detail to be worked out by Government and other appropriate organisations . . . But we foresee real dangers in the law intervening too fast and too extensively in areas where there is no clear public consensus. Furthermore both medical science and opinion within society may advance with startling rapidity . . .

List of Recommendations.
We recommend that:
   A. The licensing body and its functions.
      1. A new statutory licensing authority be established to regulate both research and those infertility services which we have recommended should be subject to control.
      2. There should be substantial lay representation on the statutory authority to regulate research and infertility services and that the chairman must be a lay person.
      3. All practitioners offering the services we have recommended should only provide these under licence, and all premises used as part of any such provision, including the provision of fresh semen and banks for the storage of frozen human eggs, semen and embryos should be licensed by the licensing body.
      4. AID should be available on a properly organised basis and subject to the licensing arrangements described in [this report], to those infertile couples for whom it might be appropriate. The provision of AID services without a licence for the purpose should be an offence.
      5. The service of IVF should continue to be available subject to the same type of licensing and inspection as we have recommended with regard to the regulation of AID.
      6. Egg donation be accepted as a recognised technique in the treatment of infertility subject to the same types of licensing and controls as we have recommended for the regulation of AID and IVF.
      7. The form of embryo donation involving donated semen and egg which are brought together in vitro be accepted as a treatment for infertility, subject to the same type of licensing and controls as we have recommended with regard to the regulation of AID, IVF and egg donation.

8. The technique of embryo donation by lavage should not be used at the present time.

9. The use of frozen eggs in therapeutic procedures should not be undertaken until research has shown that no unacceptable risk is involved. This will be a matter for review by the licensing body.

10. The clinical use of frozen embryos may continue to be developed under review by the licensing body.

11. Research conducted on human in-vitro embryos and the handling of such embryos should be permitted only under license.

12. No live human embryo derived from in-vitro fertilisation, whether frozen or unfrozen, may be kept alive, if not transferred to a woman beyond fourteen days after fertilisation, nor may it be used as a research subject beyond fourteen days after fertilisation. This fourteen-day period does not include any time during which the embryo may have been frozen.

13. Consent be obtained as to the method of use or disposal of spare embryos.

14. As a matter of good practice no research should be carried out on a spare embryo without the informed consent of the couple from whom the embryo was generated, whenever this is possible.

15. Where trans-species fertilisation is used as part of a recognised programme for alleviating infertility or in the assessment or diagnosis of sub-fertility, it should be subject to licence and that a condition of granting such a licence should be that the development of any resultant hybrid should be terminated at the two-cell stage.

16. The licensing body be asked to consider the need for follow-up studies of children born as a result of the new techniques, including consideration of the need for a centrally maintained register of such births.

17. The sale or purchase of human gametes or embryos should be permitted only under licence, from and subject to, conditions prescribed by the licensing body.

B. Principles of provision.

18. As a matter of good practice any third party donating

gametes for infertility treatment should be unknown to the couple before, during and after the treatment, and equally the third party should not know the identity of the couple being helped.

19. Counselling should be available to all infertile couples and third parties at any stage of the treatment, both as an integral part of NHS provision and in the private sector.

20. In the case of more specialised forms of infertility treatment the consent in writing of both partners should be obtained, wherever possible, before treatment is begun, as a matter of good practice. Any written consent should be obtained on an appropriate consent form.

21. The formal consent in writing by both partners should, as a matter of good practice, always be obtained before AID treatment begins. A consent form should be used and thoroughly explained to both partners.

22. For the present, there should be a limit of ten children who can be fathered by one donor.

23. In cases where consultants decline to provide treatment they should always give the patient a full explanation of the reasons.

24. The NHS numbers of all donors be checked by the clinics where they make their donations against a new centrally maintained list of NHS numbers of existing donors, which is to be held separately from the NHS donor register.

25. There should be a gradual move towards a system where semen donors should be given only their expenses.

26. In relation to egg donation the principles of good practice we have already considered in relation to other techniques should apply, including the anonymity of the donor, limitation of the number of children born from the eggs of any one donor to ten, openness with the child about his genetic origins, the availability of counselling for all parties, and informed consent.

27. It should be accepted practice to offer donated gametes and embryos to those at risk of transmitting hereditary disorders.

28. All types of 'do-it-yourself' sex selection kits should be brought within the ambit of control provided by the

Medicines Act with the aim of ensuring that such products are safe, efficacious and of an acceptable standard for use.

29. The use of frozen semen in artificial insemination should continue.

30. There should be automatic five-yearly reviews of semen and egg deposits.

31. There should be a maximum of ten years for the storage of embryos, after which time the right to use or disposal should pass to the storage authority.

32. When one of a couple dies the right to use or dispose of any embryo stored by that couple should pass to the survivor. If both die that right should pass to the storage authority.

33. Where there is no agreement between the couple the right to determine the use or disposal of an embryo should pass to the storage authority as though the ten-year period had expired.

C. Service provision.

34. Funding should be made available for the collection of adequate statistics on infertility and infertility services.

35. Each health authority should review its facilities for the investigation and treatment of infertility and consider the establishment, separate from routine gynaecology, of a specialist infertility clinic with close working relationships with specialist units, including genetic counselling services, at regional and supra-regional level.

36. Where it is not possible to have a separate clinic, infertility patients should be seen separately from other types of gynaecology patient, wherever possible.

37. The establishment of a working group at national level be made up of central health departments, health authorities and those working in infertility, to draw up detailed guidance on the organisation of services.

38. Consideration be given to the inclusion of plans for infertility services as part of the next round of health authority strategic plans.

39. IVF should continue to be available within the NHS.

40. One of the first tasks of the working group, whose establishment we recommend (above), should be to

consider how best an IVF service can be organised within the NHS.

D. Legal limits on research.

41. The embryo of the human species should be afforded some protection in law.

42. Any unauthorised use of an in-vitro embryo would in itself constitute a criminal offence.

43. Legislation should provide that research may be carried out on any embryo resulting from in-vitro fertilisation, whatever its provenance, up to the end of the fourteenth day after fertilisation, but subject to all other restrictions as may be imposed by the licensing body.

44. It shall be a criminal offence to handle or to use as a research subject any live human embryo derived from in-vitro fertilisation beyond that limit (i.e., fourteen days after fertilisation).

45. No embryo which has been used for research should be transferred to a woman.

46. Any unlicensed uses of sub-species fertilisation involving human gametes should be a criminal offence.

47. The placing of a human embryo in the uterus of another species for gestation should be a criminal offence.

48. The proposed licensing body promulgate guidance on what types of research, apart from those precluded by law, would be unlikely to be considered ethically acceptable in any circumstances and therefore would not be licensed.

49. Unauthorised sale or purchase of human gametes or embryos should be made a criminal offence.

E. Legal changes.

50. The AID child should in law be treated as the legitimate child of its mother and her husband, where they have both consented to the treatment.

51. A change in the law so that the semen donor will have no parental rights or duties in relation to the child.

52. Following the English Law Commission, that it should be presumed that the husband has consented to AID, unless the contrary is proved.

53. The law should be changed so as to permit the husband to be registered as the father.

54.  Legislation should provide that when a child is born of a woman following donation of another's egg the woman giving birth should, for all purposes, be regarded in law as the mother of that child, and that the egg donor should have no rights or obligations in respect of the child.

55.  The legislation proposed in recommendations 53 and 54 should cover children born following embryo donation.

56.  Legislation should be introduced to render criminal the creation or the operation in the United Kingdom of agencies whose purposes include the recruitment of women for surrogate pregnancy or making arrangements for individuals or couples who wish to utilise the services of a carrying mother; such legislation should be wide enough to include both profit and non-profit making organisations.

57.  Legislation should be sufficiently wide to render criminally liable the actions of professionals and others who knowingly assist in the establishment of a surrogate pregnancy.

58.  It is provided by statute that all surrogacy agreements are illegal contracts and therefore unenforceable in the courts.

59.  Legislation should provide that where a person dies during the storage period or cannot be traced at a review date, the right of use or disposal of his or her frozen gametes should pass to the storage authority.

60.  Legislation be introduced to provide that any child born by AID who was not in utero at the date of the death of its father shall be disregarded for the purposes of succession to and inheritance from the latter.

61.  Legislation be enacted to ensure there is no right of ownership in a human embryo.

62.  For the purpose of establishing primogeniture the date and time of birth and not the date of fertilisation shall be the determining factor.

63.  Legislation be introduced to provide that any child born following IVF, using an embryo that had been frozen and stored, who was not in utero at the date of the death of the father shall be disregarded for the purposes of succession to and inheritance from the latter.

It would not be useful for me to comment here on the Warnock Committee's findings in any great detail. At the time of their appearance they were widely perceived as being very liberal: virtually all professional organisations in science and medicine supported them, while every instrument of reactionary lay conservatism rose instantly up in arms against them. To me, however, the report's emphasis on the criminalisation of certain actions seemed needlessly repressive: 'one of society's bluntest instruments . . . what business is it of the law to be interfering at all?' one distinguished lawyer, A.T.H. Smith, agreed. Regulation was necessary, certainly, and a fourteen-day limit on embryo research was for some people a reasonable guiding principle, but Warnock created for me the unsuitable image of policemen standing by in research laboratories, their stopwatches poised, as the hour of midnight on the fourteenth day approached. And anyway, why should embryo research become suddenly illegal with the striking of a clock when open-ended research on the tissues of abortuses at twenty weeks of pregnancy could take place freely? And on the matter of surrogacy, it seemed to me odd that public surrogacy should be considered wrong when it was accepted in private.

Still, the Warnock Committee's report represented a sincere attempt to focus well-informed public debate, and it promised to provide a sound basis for legislation for Parliament by the Government's Department of Health and Social Security.

The report lifted heavy ethical obligations from my shoulders. Before this, Patrick and I had stood first in the firing line, initiating and doing the work, and justifying it, and now Dame Mary would take that responsibility. 'Celebrations were in order at Dr Robert Edwards's embryo laboratory in Cambridge at the weekend,' concluded Andrew Veitch of the *Guardian* on 18 June 1984. He was certainly right. 'If the main recommendations of the Warnock Committee are accepted, Britain will become the most liberal country in the world as far as work on human embryos is concerned.'

Much vehement, if inconclusive wordage, has flowed under various parliamentary bridges during the five years since the report was published. It now seems (in October 1988) that a lot more will have to flow before the British Government takes decisive action either to accept or reject the committee's recommendations.

# 8
# The Lawyers

It is notoriously difficult to frame meaningful laws concerning the sexual vagaries, or the reproductive hopes and fears of men and women. It is also usually pointless: no matter what, people will continue to make their own decisions about their fertility or sexuality. Lesbians determined to conceive, for example, will obtain semen somehow, whatever the law may say. Women wishing to abort their fetuses can be equally determined: in some Latin American countries where laws against abortion have been strict, so many back-street operators come to practise that blood banks in the cities become depleted as doctors try to save the illegally aborted mothers from bleeding to death. And when, as in Communist China, laws to control population growth restrict families to one child each, so powerful is the traditional need for a son that, as the *Economist* reported in 1983, 'In 1980 and 1981 forty girl babies were drowned in one village . . . Midwives in Guamgdom, according to local newspapers, plunge a girl baby straight into a bucket of water . . . and simply record a stillbirth.'

Most governments recognise their basic powerlessness in such matters. They prefer to limit legislation to narrow, particular issues, and even then — as in the case of commercial surrogacy in Britain — only act when public or legal pressure leave them no alternative. Lawyers and judges, therefore, mostly find themselves obliged to handle potential litigation on a piecemeal basis, on its merits as and when it arises, and must rely principally on precedent — which is a risky business in these days of unforeseen possibilities and unimaginably rapid change.

In 1938 a London physician, Dr Bourne, was approached by colleagues asking him to perform an abortion on a pregnant fourteen-year-old girl who had been raped by a number of soldiers. Although laws on abortion were obscure at the time, governed principally by the Offences Against the Person Act of 1861 or the Infant Life Preservation Act of 1929, Dr Bourne was aware that he would risk prosecution if he performed the operation. But he had discreetly aborted similar cases before, so in the interests of the patient he decided to do so again — only on this occasion, in order to establish a test case and clarify the law, he announced the date and the time of the abortion and was duly brought to trial for performing an illegal operation. Justice Macnaghten was the presiding judge; he found the abortion to have been justified in the circumstances, and Dr Bourne was acquitted.

This proved to be a very influential judgment, and it led by slow degrees to the easing of abortion laws both here in Britain and in other countries.

Pioneers willing to face imprisonment have come forward similarly in the field of contraception. In Victorian times Annie Besant and the MP Charles Bradlaugh were tried and found guilty of obscenity — their crime had been to offer pamphlets on family planning to the British working classes. It was a trial that back-fired, however: the two offenders' sentences were later commuted on technical grounds, and the resulting publicity had meanwhile greatly increased the sales of their contraception literature.

In America, even in the twentieth century, the women's activist Margaret Sanger was less fortunate. She was jailed several times in New York for teaching women how to control their own fertility.

Hindsight, by undermining our respect for past laws, often encourages us to be sceptical of laws in general. But disregard for the law in medical matters is not always ethically straightforward. The American scientist Gregory Pincus may be admired for having developed the first contraceptive pill, but his early tests were only possible because they were performed on Puerto Rican women who were less well protected by law than his fellow Americans. And how do we feel when our governments authorise monstrous bacteriological weapons ostensibly for our protection, or when astronauts walk on the moon by courtesy of German engineers using knowledge gained through illegal and inhumane research in Nazi concentration camps?

And how do we feel, also, when developments in embryology raise the spectre of human babies being regarded merely as means to an end, rather than as ends in themselves? Such cases have already arisen in America where couples conceived a child for spare parts for their existing child. Another mother strove to bring her anencephalic fetus – a fetus so drastically malformed as to be virtually without a brain – to full term simply in order that those of its organs that were normal could be used at its birth for transplants.

The case raised considerable outcry, but ethical difficulties were to be evaded by keeping the baby alive on a respirator until it died naturally, and the procedure was too novel for the law to have developed anything useful to say in the matter. In the event, the fetus solved everyone's problems by being stillborn. But the law, either in the US or here in Britain, remains powerless to stop other individuals from obtaining – or perhaps even commissioning – plentiful supplies of graft material and donor organs from non-viable fetuses brought unnaturally to birth. Indeed, heart transplants have already been done using tissues from fetuses found to be anencephalic at birth.

The difficulty is clear. When each one of us has strong positive opinions on a particular issue, we expect the lawyers to intervene on our behalf, such as those husbands filing suits against their wives who abort their fetus without their consent, but in all other cases we prefer the law to remain tactfully impotent. In 1983 a baby girl was born with Down's syndrome in Indiana. Since her parents felt unable to cope with this handicap and she also suffered from an intestinal obstruction which threatened her life, they refused their permission for a surgical operation to clear the obstruction. The child eventually died. Although her case received much publicity in the USA at the time and calls were made for changes in a law that might be said to permit, by a positive act of refusal, the wilful murder of an infant, no such changes have so far been made, or indeed seem likely in the future. This has not been the first example of such a birth. And underlying all decisions concerning such cases are the future prospects for happiness of any child so profoundly unwanted by its guilt-ridden and unhappy parents.

After all, lawyers when sufficiently pressed are often able to stretch the provisions of existing laws to make them apply. In New York, in 1978, a couple sued the Columbia Presbyterian Medical Center when an embryo of theirs, conceived in vitro, was thrown down the drain. A doctor at the hospital had apparently set up the fertilisation in good faith but his professor doubted his ability and feared that the embryo would be abnormal, and anyway the hospital's ethical committee on experimentation had not approved the work, so the embryo was taken from its culture dish and simply discarded.

Its parents were upset. They sued for damages, for denial of the right to have a child, and for emotional distress, and they won. They were awarded $50,000 for the emotional distress, but nothing for the loss of their embryo. Nor was there any mention of wrongful death since in the United States and elsewhere lawyers apply this concept only to a person, and in law *personhood* only occurs at birth: until a fetus has been born alive it is simply a thing in their eyes, its mother's property, her chattel.

The lawyers' judgment may seem simplistic in view of the ethnical maze non-lawyers build round the matter, but it has the singular virtue of limiting scope for future litigation. If an embryo were considered a person in law, then the conflict of rights between a woman and the embryo in her womb could lead to unending legal disputes. She might be compelled by it to live in a certain way, not to drink or smoke, perhaps, in order to minimise the risks of damage to it. And the legality of all abortions would be in serious doubt if embryos and fetuses ceased to be legally regarded simply as chattels.

Which is not to say that the law, perhaps with faulty logic, does not grant certain rights to these fetuses. If they are born alive, they can inherit their dead fathers' estates. Also, once born, they can be compensated for injuries caused to them in their mothers' wombs. A Montreal court was the first to grant such compensation, in 1933, after a pregnant woman had fallen from a tramcar. Her baby was born injured and the tramway company was ordered to compensate both mother and child. It was a decision widely adopted across the USA and Europe, but there was a significant reservation: the child had to be born alive. Compensation has been awarded to children who are scarred as a fetus by a chemical or hormone, the careless use of a knife, by a remedy improperly administered or a condition improperly diagnosed — but very few fetuses which have died in utero after the moment of viability have made a successful claim in US courts, no matter who or what has caused their deaths.

This is a complex area of law, full of uncertainties centring on who has caused the damage, the cause itself, and the rights of the fetuses. Responsibilities are blurred, for example, in cases concerning accidental infections, or medicines administered before conception or where the woman did not know she was pregnant. But penalties *have* been imposed against a doctor for performing an incorrect blood transfusion years before a handicapped child was born, and against another in favour of a child born severely damaged after the doctor had failed to test its mother properly for German measles. Parents have been sued for a child's illegitimacy, and also when one or other of them has had syphilis or some other disease which has injured their fetus. And a child born with Tay-Sachs disease was awarded damages in California in 1980 against a testing laboratory which failed to identify its condition while it was still a fetus and could have been aborted. (Tay-Sachs, a disease which is characterised by neurological degeneration, invariably brings about death in early childhood.)

In Britain the thalidomide disaster stimulated legislation in 1976 which penalises anyone causing injury to a child while it is in the womb, and even if the damage occurs before fertilisation. The child has to live for forty-eight hours before it can make its claim, and a case against its own mother will only be pursued in the most extreme circumstances. Since it is almost impossible to prove the cause of such damage, especially that arising before fertilisation, I wonder how many successful cases will ever be brought under this Act.

Parents can claim against bad medical advice or other causes which lead to the birth of a damaged child. This has become known as wrongful birth, and in one US case parents have been compensated for emotional distress and for the costs of raising a sick child because their physicians had failed to warn them that it might suffer from a genetic disorder.

Very occasionally, the child itself severely damaged at birth can bring perhaps the most tragic claim of all, that of wrongful life. A child pleads that it would be better dead, would have been better aborted than born at all, that its life is a disaster, hopeless even before it began.

A grossly malformed child was born in the USA in 1967 after its mother had contracted German measles during her pregnancy. It sued its doctor for wrongful life, claiming that its parents would have aborted it had they been told the full implications of the disease. The judges made their decision: 'The infant plaintiff would have us measure the difference between his life with defects, against the utter void of non-existence. But it is impossible to make such a determination. This court cannot weigh the value of life with impairments against the non-existence of life itself.'

More recently, in 1981, a similar case was brought in Pennsylvania, which met with a similar judgment: 'Whether it is better to have never been born at all, rather than to have been born with serious mental defects, is a mystery more properly left to the philosophers and theologians, a mystery which would lead us into the field of metaphysics, beyond the realm of our understanding or ability to solve.'

In Britain, a year later, Judge Ackner was equally firm: 'But how can a court begin to evaluate non-existence, the undiscovered country from whose bourne no traveller returns? No comparison is possible and therefore no damage can be established which a court could recognise.'

Lawyers feel on safer ground when defending a couple's right to bear children — and with good reason, since the right to found a family is written into declarations both from the United Nations Assembly and from the European Court of Law. The US Supreme Court too, in accepting the individual's right to privacy, has granted that this includes the couple's right to conceive children: 'If the right to privacy means anything, it is the right of the individual, married or single, to be free from unwarranted government intrusion into matters so fundamentally affecting a person as the decision whether to bear or beget a child.'

The same legislatures that defend the individual's right to bear children also become more sure of themselves once the children have been born. In Britain in 1968 a baby born in Berkshire was found to be addicted to drugs taken by its mother, so the County Council removed it from her care and placed it in the charge of foster parents. The mother took her case on appeal as high as the House of Lords, but lost both it and her baby. And in the same year, in

California, another woman's behaviour during pregnancy was seen as affecting her rights once her child had been born. She had taken amphetamines while pregnant, her child was born brain-damaged, and it died shortly afterwards. Accused of contributing to her son's death by her drug-taking, she faced charges of manslaughter, but was acquitted.

The law is now moving back to involve itself in the earliest stages of conception or even before, and stands poised like the Sword of Damocles over doctors and scientists practising in-vitro fertilisation. No wonder our sponsors pulled out from Bourn Hall in 1980! More than fifty women were infected with viral hepatitis in a Dutch clinic, the fault of a serum used to grow embryos. In the United States a child, conceived in vitro, has apparently been born of the wrong father. Legal action is possible in both these cases. And legal threats worry doctors replacing too many embryos, and risking quintuplets or more and then having to reduce the pregnancy by selectively aborting two or three. In many countries, the law will also deal with the status of embryos in vitro and research on them. In Germany, it seems certain that among other items, the creation of embryos purely for research will be forbidden, and the same could well happen in France.

Arguably lawyers and judges are not to be blamed when their responses to the reproduction revolution seem confused or inconsistent. Some people may claim that the law has a duty to lead society, to guide it through today's ethical minefields, but in general the law is seen as simply underpinning the consensus. As the British solicitor, Sir David Napley, has written: 'The law, in any country, exists to protect rights . . . such as have been established by Parliament or any other law-giving authority, or which have been recognised under the Common Law . . . as having so long existed and been so long recognised that they cannot now be gainsaid . . . [Courts] never make new law but merely declare what the law . . . has been.'

And certainly the confusions of the laws surrounding embryology and assisted reproduction today are no more than a reflection of the confusions of a society in which the consensus has completely broken down. The influential American lawyer, Katheryn Lorio, may well write that 'the absence of any consensus as to the propriety of the [medical] procedure indicates the need for some general guidelines', but I know she would be the first to agree that in any democracy such guidelines must reasonably be expected to come not from the lawyers but from the elected politicians. And these elected politicians, buffetted to and fro over the last few years by the vagaries of public opinion and the uncertainty of their own often ill-informed convictions, have found themselves as low on guidelines as everybody else.

Presumably many new and passionate arguments about the rights of embryos at conception must have been raised in Britain in the eighteenth century, when John Hunter carried out the first human artificial insemination. Certainly the dispute has gone on ever since, with debates in Britain in the early years of this century, and a Canadian court fretting about it in 1921. More recently, in 1948, the Church of England's Society for the Propagation of Christian Knowledge considered donor insemination and decided that, '. . . artificial insemination with donated semen involves a breach of the marriage. It violates the exclusive union set up between husband and wife . . . We therefore judge artificial insemination with donated semen to be wrong in principle and contrary to Christian standards . . . The evils involved . . . are so grave that early consideration should be given to the framing of legislation to make the practice a criminal offence.'

The government dragged its feet, however, waiting to see what happened. And what happened was that donor insemination was widely welcomed, increased, and gained respectability until, in 1973, the British Medical Association was able to recommend that it became available within the National Health Service.

Meanwhile, in the USA today lawyers defend their clients' rights to such technology. In Sweden and Germany laws are passed on behalf of the child, insisting that it must know the name of the donor when it reaches the age of eighteen, whereas Norway, just over their borders, requires that the name of the donor shall be permanently secret.

And still, in Britain and many other countries, no formal laws exist to control the donation of sperm, eggs, or embryos. Even the British law forbidding the recipient's husband from registering as the child's father is universally ignored: parents see no reason to record on a public document the intimate details of their child's conception, either for its future sake or for their own, and who can honestly blame them?

We look for guidelines here, and in many other areas of the reproduction revolution, but the government prefers to temporise. One can only wonder for how much longer this unsatisfactory situation will be allowed to continue.

# 9
# Surrogacy

Any discussion on the ethics of IVF would be incomplete without considering surrogate pregnancy. Like abortion, childbirth by proxy has been around for a long time. But, unlike abortion, it has been widely approved for centuries. Evidence from the Bible shows that even the Jews, a tribe that practised strict monogamy, would accept surrogacy if the social or emotional need for a child were great enough. 'Abram's wife Sara had not born him any children. But she had an Egyptian slave-girl named Hagar, so she said to Abram, "The Lord has kept me from having children. Why don't you sleep with my slave-girl? Perhaps she can have a child for me."'

Later on in Genesis, Rachel too, if for less admirable reasons, proposes surrogacy: 'but Rachel had not born Jacob any children, and so she became jealous of her sister and said to Jacob, "Give me children or I will die . . . Here is my slave-girl Bilhah: sleep with her so that she can have a child for me."' (*The Good News Bible*, Today's English Version.)

Even in those days there may well have been one set of standards for the rich and another for the poor: a society's moral strictures usually bear less heavily upon the rulers than upon the ruled. But it seems safe to assume that all down history, if a woman were barren and either she or her husband wanted children badly enough, the obvious alternative of a surrogate child-bearer might discreetly have been employed. On any scale of evils childlessness was surely far greater than the tactful flouting of a few marriage laws.

And that is the role of the surrogate mother, as a biologically straightforward remedy for a couple's childlessness. She offers her reproductive ability for conception and gestation only, denying any intention of keeping the child. Today, although some men still establish the pregnancy as in the past, by committing adultery, most surrogate mothers are artificially inseminated with spermatozoa from the commissioning husband. But in either case the surrogate conceives her own child, and then gives it away. This is not a course to be lightly undertaken, but it has a tradition of respectability — often between sisters, out of love, but also between master and servant, out of duty.

Such surrogate pregnancies have recently made big headlines. This is neither because our consciences have suddenly become more delicate, nor is it particularly because of advances in the science of embryology. It is rather because of unfettered commercialism and the growing presence of lawyers and media men and women in even the most private areas of our lives.

At first glance commercial surrogacy by artificial insemination seems a minefield of ethical difficulties. It is widely practised in the US, evidently organised by lawyers as well as by doctors. One American lawyer, Herbert T. Krimmel, tells us: 'To sanction the use and treatment of human beings as means to the achievement of other goals instead of as ends in themselves is to accept an ethic with a dangerous past, and to establish a precedent with a dangerous future. Already the press has reported the decision of one couple to conceive a child for the purpose of using it as a bone marrow donor for its sibling.'

Commercial surrogacy also smacks of the production line, and of avarice as babies are manufactured for cash, sometimes for large amounts — more than £13,000 for one attempt in Britain in 1984, $20,000 and more in the USA.

Public outrage is inflamed by the behaviour of certain baby agencies, and serious fears are felt that the reality of many women conceiving children they do not themselves want may fundamentally change and downgrade the way all of us look at children.

Further ethical problems loom once a surrogate pregnancy has produced the required baby. No matter for what reason the pregnancy was undertaken, it can be argued that birth is the foundation point of parenthood, the only necessary proof of any mother–child relationship, and the irrevocable moment when bonding between mother and child takes place. Barbara Cohen, herself a surrogate mother, writes in the *American Journal of Law and Medicine*: '[I had been] naive to think that [I] could keep from being attached to the child . . . even though I told myself again and again during the pregnancy that it was really not my baby.'

In commercial surrogacy, then, what should be done about the surrogate mother who changes her mind once the baby is born and decides to keep it? As much as any woman's it is 'her' child – should money, or a previous signature on a dotted line have any bearing on a decision so basic and elemental?

On the other hand, if the commissioning couple change their minds, perhaps because the baby has been born abnormal, should they be compelled to keep it? And keep it whether the anomaly arose in sperm or egg, or even if, as has already tragically been the case, the child suffers from an illness such as fetal alcohol syndrome, the direct consequence of the surrogate mother's unsuspected heavy drinking? After all, it is the husband's offspring, even if it is not the wife's. What can be the prospects for a child forced on to reluctant commissioning parents in such circumstances? In another case an AIDS-infected baby has been born of a surrogate mother who contracted the disease while pregnant. What should be the commissioning parents' obligations then?

Serious though these difficulties are, they seem to me

finally to be matters for law, put to the service of common sense, rather than for ethics. There must be a point where law takes over, and surely the law has had enough time to consider surrogacy! In any case, once the pregnancy is over, commercial or otherwise, it must always be the child's interests that prevail. And society has long agreed to trust judges and courts of law ultimately in such matters.

As to the ethical position of the commercial surrogate mother, this too seems to me straightforward. In the past women have accepted surrogate pregnancies for many different reasons − from obedience to a master, through simple generosity and love, to a wish for the sheer pleasure in being pregnant that some of them experience.

There is nothing scientifically novel about any of this. Artificial insemination and IVF are standardised now, so the challenge of surrogacy does not lie in novel research or complicated techniques, rather it lies in deciding the status of a uterine mother, and, of course, all the other implications of hiring her service.

Emotive phrases are brandished − like rent-a-womb − and titillating stories abound. Lord Denning, in 1986, told the House of Lords: 'A man . . . had married a lady a good deal older than himself . . . [who] would not or could not have [a child]. They went along to Bow Street and found a prostitute who acted as a go-between . . . a girl of nineteen should be artificially inseminated with the husband's semen . . .' The House was duly outraged.

Similarly, if less understandably, the British Medical Association has recently been reported in *The Times* as concluding that 'the interests of [infertile] couples are outweighed by legitimate social conditions.' I can't honestly see why. Do these doctors consider 'legitimate social conditions' before they swap kidneys or bone marrow between consenting adults? It seems unlikely.

Nor can I see why a woman who is willing to bear a child for another should not be paid for the service. 'There is no reason for a woman who volunteers to be a surrogate to feel downgraded or dehumanised,' writes Michael Lockwood, an Oxford philosopher, 'where she actually identifies with the end, and derives satisfaction from the thought that she is bringing happiness to another couple. There are those who think that the mere fact that money changes hands somehow puts the whole enterprise beyond the pale. But, soberly regarded, that is surely an over-reaction.' This is especially true if the surrogate has to make efforts to conceive – her chance in any one cycle is only 25 per cent anyway.

Certainly there are members of the women's liberation movement, those most likely to be intelligently concerned, who have no doubts about surrogacy's value. Mary Kenny wrote recently in the *Sunday Telegraph* that by providing choice and unfettered contractual freedom in reproduction, 'surrogacy will be the greatest extension of liberty since the abolition of slavery. Women's lives will not be unequivocally our own until pregnancy is fully under our control.'

And the record so far, in countries where commercial surrogacy by artificial insemination is regularly practised, is not at all bad. The vast majority of commissioned babies are conceived, carried, born and handed over straightforwardly, to the complete satisfaction of all concerned. Perhaps the surrogate mother does not 'bond' to her child because she intended, before it was conceived, to hand it over. Or perhaps bonding might not be important for her.

There are exceptions, inevitably, and the more outrageous these are, the more publicity they receive. One surrogate mother refused to part with the baby because she had discovered that the commissioning mother wasn't in her opinion a proper woman – having only recently become one after a sex change operation. And there was a case, resolved disgracefully, in the shoddy glare of a television chat show, in which a mentally subnormal child was able to be rejected by the commissioning parents because paternity tests showed it was not the child of the commissioning husband.

There is a dark side, also, to the work of surrogate agencies. They have been paid by the commissioning couple, they have a contract with the surrogate mother, and if they do not get the agreed baby they may feel obliged to try to enforce the law by every possible means. This is not an edifying spectacle. Neither is it edifying when intrusive journalists are tipped off by an agency or someone else, ferret out a surrogate mother, and hound her all through her pregnancy until the moment when, to the clicking of cameras, she finally hands over the new-born child.

Any surrogate pregnancy is a nail-biting time for the agency. The surrogate mother may conceive deceitfully by another man to make sure of her money, abort either spontaneously or even deliberately for she has this right under law, she may take drugs, she may disappear on a long holiday, get married, or even attempt a sort of blackmail as the months go by, by trying to raise the stakes. The commissioning couple, too, cannot be relied on. They may change their minds – perhaps because they have un-expectedly conceived a child of their own, or perhaps because the husband has suddenly lost his job and is penniless. They may separate or divorce . . . They may both die in a car crash, so that the child is an orphan even before it is born. In the face of so many uncertainties, it is hardly surprising that some agencies are less than tactful in their initial checking procedures, and oppressive in their subsequent surveillance.

But after all this is said, I still do not believe that any of these issues are ethical in character. They are matters for the law. I may not envy the law-makers their task, but I place all questions concerning conventional commercial surrogacy squarely upon their table. If all the parties employing an adoption agency can be protected, as is now the case, then so can all the parties involved with a surrogacy agency.

Only one major problem needs to be solved: the legal validity of a surrogacy contract. In some countries, for example, to pay a woman to hand over a child might be considered the making of a payment to induce an adoption or to buy a child, both generally unacceptable in law. It might even offend anti-slavery laws. Or if surrogacy could be held contrary to public policy, then all arrangements between surrogates, agencies and commissioning parents would not be legally enforceable.

This should be no great drawback, however; usually, when a case gets to court there are factors other than the contract on which judges can base their decisions. In the 1986 Baby M case in New Jersey, Mr and Mrs Stern had employed a surrogate, Mrs Whitehead, who bore a child through artificial insemination with Mr Stern's spermatozoa. Mrs Whitehead then became attached to the child, refused the $10,000 fee, and fled with the baby. She was found in Florida. The Sterns wished to claim the child as their own, and insisted on the validity of their contract with Mrs Whitehead, so the case was brought to court.

The publicity was enormous, the reporting generally offensive. Mrs Stern had chosen surrogacy because she suffered from multiple sclerosis − now it was suggested, quite irrelevantly, that her disease was not sufficiently advanced to preclude pregnancy and that she had only sought a surrogate because she wanted a baby but didn't want to interrupt her career. On the other side, Mrs Whitehead's qualifications as a mother were criticised also − she had worked as a bar-room dancer and her life with her husband Richard had been marked by instability.

The judge found in favour of the Sterns, granting them custody of the child. But he made it clear that he was doing so entirely in its interests, and not as a judgment on the legality of the surrogacy contract. Mrs Whitehead then took her case to a higher court. She felt that she had been discriminated against on account of her former career as a dancer, her hairstyle, and her taste in children's toys, and she gained many supporters including an organisation of distinguished American women. 'By these standards we are all unfit mothers . . . We strongly urge legislators and jurors . . . to recognise that a mother need not be perfect to deserve her child.' The basic strength of Mrs Whitehead's argument was not undermined when she later found herself pregnant.

The appeal court in New Jersey modified the judge's decision, awarding custody of the child to Mr Stern because Mrs Whitehead was not fit, but removing parental rights from Mrs Stern and reinstating Mrs Whitehead as the natural mother, thus granting her access to the child. So that it seems to have been humanity, and the interests of the child, that won through finally, even in this extreme case of a troubled conventional commercial surrogacy.

Nevertheless, some American states have legislated against surrogacy, and two reporters on the *Washington Post*, N.J. Meiselman and T.M. Schuch, point out that a woman bearing a child is its natural mother until she relinquishes her rights through adoption. Any child conceived and born in marriage is the legitimate issue of both spouses, they stress, referring to a decision by Lord Mansfield in 1777, so Mr Stern's fertilising sperm could be considered a gift to the Whiteheads, and in that case Richard Whitehead was clearly the legal father (*Washington Post*, 22 September 1987). I firmly believe though, that this tortuous argument can never alter the biological fact that Mr Stern was the genetic father of the child.

Today, surrogacy can be done in a totally different way. A commissioning couple can conceive their own embryo in vitro provided the wife has eggs in her ovary. It does not matter if she is over forty, if her womb is becoming too old to gestate a fetus, or if she has no womb at all. It is possible for an embryo to be flushed from her womb and placed in a surrogate mother, who now has no genetic or familial relationship whatsoever to any child that may be born. She is merely the uterine mother, and nothing else.

Different questions are raised by what I will call 'host' surrogacy. Today every imaginable permutation of egg, sperm and womb has been made possible by in-vitro fertilisation, coupled with advances in embryo research. A fertile woman who for some reason cannot carry a child — perhaps she has no womb — can have her egg fertilised in vitro by her husband's sperm, or a donor's, and the resulting embryo can be implanted in a surrogate mother. By means of host surrogacy, therefore, even a woman perfectly healthy in every way can choose, perhaps for professional or cosmetic reasons, to employ surrogates to bear her children. Now the surrogate is totally unrelated genetically to the child — she is simply the uterine mother. This may largely dispose of one legal question constantly raised about surrogacy by artificial insemination, that parents may not 'barter or sell their children', but an American commentator, B.K Rothman, writing in *USA Today*, has suggested one possible ugly consequence of this: 'Now that surrogate mothers no longer need to be white to have white babies, the door is opened for the serious exploitation of young poor women of colour . . . "rented wombs" for the growing of expensive white babies.'

Additionally, since fertilised eggs can now be frozen and stored as embryos virtually indefinitely, a surrogate need not carry an embryo received directly from the commissioning couple: she can just as easily carry a frozen–thawed embryo from an embryo bank, the issue, perhaps, of a dead wife or lover.

A preposterous scenario? Not if some great estate or some sufficiently powerful emotion were at stake, for modern genetic tests can prove the identity of an embryonic inheritor beyond all doubt. Already spermatozoa have been donated to a couple so that they could have the donor's child and raise it under his trust fund, with him acting as an uncle to it. And already in South Africa embryos from a daughter have been implanted in her mother's womb and the older woman, out of love for her, has born her daughter's triplets. What price the laws of inheritance now, or the dictionary definition of a mother as 'a woman who has borne a child'?

A judge in Wayne, Michigan, has already faced this last problem. Ruling in a case concerning the maternity and paternity rights to a child born of a surrogate mother by way of embryo transfer, Judge Marianne O. Battani gave this opinion:

We really have no definition of *mother* in our law . . . It is important to recognise the intent of the parties in this situation . . . I am limiting my opinion to the circumstances of this case, where the parties first contracted to do this . . . where there is an in-vitro fertilisation and where it can be confirmed by paternity—maternity testing that the implanted ovum is in fact the child that resulted from the in-vitro fertilisation . . . I do make a determination that the donor of the ovum, the biological mother, is to be deemed in fact the natural mother of this infant, as is the biological father to be deemed the natural father of this child.

The judge therefore ordered that the name of the mother written on the birth certificate should be that of the biological mother; for the first time in western legal history the facts of the conception of a child were considered more important than the facts of its birth. Genetics had triumphed over physiology!

Back in 1970, when Patrick Steptoe and I had made our first break-through in in-vitro fertilisation, we discussed many allied possibilities. 'What about surrogacy for some of your patients?' I asked him one morning in the laboratory. 'It shouldn't be difficult, now that the embryos are growing in vitro so well.'

He frowned. 'Let's think about that after we've managed to get a few babies. I've got thousands of patients eager to bear their own children. Let's wait until we've helped them before we start worrying about surrogacy.'

At that time we could put off the decision. I no longer can. At present commercial surrogacy is illegal in Britain, but I frequently attend and speak at seminars in other countries, including the USA and France, where doctors use it regularly, and my belief is that surrogacy will ultimately become acceptable, provided that careful counselling is available for all concerned, surrogates, couples and perhaps even doctors and embryologists, to make sure the procedure is fully understood. It's easy for those of us with our children growing up happily around us to feel distaste for the booming business of the surrogacy agencies, to feel dismay at the potential for litigation that surrogacy brings with it, and to feel anxiety for the happiness of the children that are the movement's justification. But very similar problems were once faced over adoption. And court battles over surrogacy should not be over-emphasised; similar legal strife arose in the early days of contraception, donor insemination, abortion and fetal screening.

There have always been pregnancies by surrogacy and there always will be. They do not necessarily lead to ethical problems and they can be a great blessing. The introduction of payment as a factor raises legal questions but leaves the ethics unchanged. Perhaps it may be thought less worthy to perform an act for money rather than for love, but it is hardly wrong.

As to the disasters, most of these can be eliminated by care and foresight. Agencies can be made subject to regulation, to licensing and to strict supervision. The best intermediary might be a State Board: this would set fees, encourage volunteers and negotiate between commissioning couple and surrogate, rigorously screening both.

Should Patrick and I have undertaken surrogate pregnancies back in the seventies, giving many parents their own children instead of letting them gradually lose all hope as their infertility became final in the menopause? Yes, we should have, provided that it could have been done under wise and compassionate supervision.

'When Leah realised she had stopped having children, she gave her slave-girl Zilpah to Jacob as his wife. And Zilpah bore Jacob a son . . .' Perhaps this is a case where the Bible can indeed teach us a lesson or two.

# 10
# The Politicians

In a sense the political IVF debate in Britain might be said to have begun twenty years ago, when the government, responding to medical developments and to changes in social attitudes, recognised a need to reform the then extremely strict and prohibitory British laws on abortion. The matter was much debated, both inside and outside Parliament, and eventually an Act was passed with the intention of permitting abortion in many cases of genuine need, while maintaining rigid governmental control over the criteria and the decision-making process. But the Act was loosely worded, dangerously so – and particularly in one provision which laid down that a mother could be permitted to abort her fetus in order to 'save her from greater harm'.

This was a humanely-intended phrase, but clearly the politicians who approved it were unaware that medically speaking birth could in most cases be considered a greater hazard to the mother than abortion, so that in practical terms this provision would provide an excuse for the almost unlimited termination of pregnancies. This is what actually happened. Parliament's wishes were circumvented, abortion virtually on demand became legally available, and London became the abortion capital of the world.

Over the next twenty years, as liberalising influences have spread across Europe and the USA, Britain has gradually lost its special status and doubtful attraction. Even so, British society has remained deeply divided on the subject of abortion, and repeated attempts have been made — even until today — in Parliament to recast the relevant laws. So far these have met with little success; societies in general preserve the status quo best, even if it is widely seen as unsatisfactory, and Britain is particularly good at the preservation game.

With the past mistakes of the Abortion Act very much in mind, therefore, British politicians faced with public concern over the ethics of embryology, and the need for legislation, have been intensely reluctant to commit themselves. But in 1984, when the report of the Warnock Committee was finally published, they had no further excuse for delay.

The year, incidentally, underlines the uncanny prescience of George Orwell, writing of it back in 1948: 'We have cut the link between child and parent and between man and man and between man and woman . . . Children will be taken from their mothers at birth as one takes eggs from a hen . . . The sex instincts will be a formality . . .' (*1984*, George Orwell, Penguin Books, 1949).

In any event, as pressures for action on the Warnock Report — some approving, some vengeful — built up inside and outside Parliament, the British Government proceeded cautiously. To test the water, it decided first to hold an open, non-party debate in the House of Lords. A conservative response was expected from this most antique of parliamentary chambers, but its eccentric and wildly unrepresentative membership often disappoints even the most reliable expectations.

In October 1984 a government minister rose in the House of Lords to open the debate. The government, he claimed unsurprisingly, had acted wisely and consulted widely. They did not want to be hasty in judging such complex issues of life and death.

Some Lords and Ladyships sympathised. Lord Ennals spoke first: a life-long politician, he took tactful refuge in the United Nations declaration on the right to have a family,

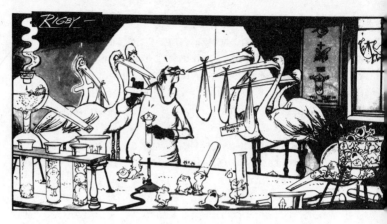

'Do you mind? Take your silent demo somewhere else!!'

which he supported. In general, therefore, he supported the Warnock Report also, since research on embryos helped this good cause, as did the donation of sperm and eggs, while surrogate motherhood was clearly quite a different, and complicated matter.

The Bishop of Chelmsford was in favour too, and accepted day 14 as the limit for research. Lord Winstanley was more cautious, but found difficulty in reconciling the Virgin Birth with recent developments in parthenogenesis.

In due course Lord Soper gave his views. I have already quoted this noble Methodist Lord in Chapter 6, but I see no harm in doing so briefly again. He pointed out that his present world was significantly different from that which had helped him fashion his moral principles, and that in making ethical judgments the Bible was only of limited assistance: 'I have to find my morality, at least in specific terms, in the process of the Christian Church . . . [Yet it] very largely lays down its principles with regard to sexual morality in terms which [are] now completely out of date and quite wrong.'

Lord Soper welcomed modern knowledge and embryo research, and was optimistic of a future where science and technology would help him to aspire to a spiritual life.

Lord Denning, a retired law lord, had predictably more mundane concerns. He wanted, primarily, to know to whom an embryo belonged. He also recommended uncompromising laws on every aspect of conception. Furthermore, since fertilisation was the only moment when life could reasonably be said to begin, fertilised eggs should be treated like children: they should not be bought or sold, experimented on or destroyed. The thought of children born of frozen embryos long after their parents were dead shocked him, if for no very clear reason, and he was astonished by the proposal that semen recipients should not know their donor, or a donor his children: never before had the law allowed a man so to evade his responsibilities.

At least Lord Denning's legal background gave him understandable reasons for resisting Warnock, for invoking the law and wishing to extend its provisions. But his words served to release a positive flood of more widely-based opposition. The Bishop of Norwich disliked most of the Warnock Report: he described himself as a defender of the principles of the ancient Judeo-Christian tradition, and he found none of them in the report. The Archbishop of Canterbury, he said, had even been right back in 1948 when he had castigated donor insemination as a criminal offence. Child or not, infertility or not, embryos must be defended and science prohibited from any intrusion. To sustain his deepest beliefs he quoted Pope John Paul II:

The world has largely lost respect for human life from the moment of conception. The world is weak in upholding the indissoluble unity of marriage. It fails to support the stability and holiness of family life. There is a crisis of truth and responsibility in human relationships. And so I support with all my heart those who recognise and defend the Law of God, which governs human life. We must never forget that every person, from the moment of conception to the last breath, is a unique child of God and has the right to life.

Other lords quickly followed the Bishop. Lord Rawlinson, a Roman Catholic, was filled with fears for the future:

he foresaw a new commandment, a moral instruction which
changed 'thou shalt not kill' to 'after an embryo has reached
fourteen days, thou *shalt* kill'. The Earl of Halsbury agreed
with him, as did the Marquess of Lothian: infertility gave
nobody the right to wield such power, no excuse to play
God.

Supporting voices clamoured to be heard. Embryos were
human: they should be protected just like other humans.
The Christian conscience must be listened to, since Jesus
Christ was incarnate by the Holy Spirit and born of the
Virgin Mary.

A few spoke up for Warnock. Lord Meston counselled
the law to caution: he suggested it play the tortoise rather
than the head-in-sand ostrich. Lord Prys-Davies, too, was
constructive: he advocated open-mindedness about research and surrogacy.

The debate ended. No vote was taken, but a majority of
the noble lords clearly disapproved of Warnock.

In the country at large, too, Warnock was in trouble. The
doctor, Professor Ian Donald, probably spelled out people's
doubts and fears very accurately when he was reported in
the *Guardian* as saying: 'We're talking about human
experimentation, not veterinary technology. A human
being has potential from the very beginning – six million
genes and all. A Frankenstein monster may not be too far
away. The dangers are very real . . . scientists are not all
saints.'

The moral watchdog LIFE organised a nationwide
petition, calling for a ban on all forms of embryo research,
and on in-vitro fertilisation too. They collected signatures,
millions of them, outside supermarkets and banks, at bus
stops and on street corners, and they encouraged their
supporters to lobby MPs against any bill on Warnock's
terms so successfully that some MPs received more anti-
research letters than the size of their considerable majorities.

In France, meanwhile, the recently established National
Ethical Committee was locked in inconclusive debate,

assessing the legitimacy of in-vitro fertilisation and the use of tissue from abortuses for transplants. In Australia the Attorney General had ruled that the ethics of embryology were a matter for each state to judge for itself, and in Victoria the influential Waller Commission had led to the legalisation of freezing and some embryo research in that state. The Scandinavian countries were actively considering the issues, and in the USA — following an unsuccessful attempt back in 1981 by the arch-conservative Senator Jesse Helms to mount a bill 'to provide that human life shall be deemed to exist from conception' (and thus incidentally overthrowing an even earlier Supreme Court ruling which had virtually legalised abortion) — Senator Albert Gore was holding preliminary hearings on the matter.

Clearly the problem wasn't going to go away. So, as public pressure became too great to resist, the British Government acted again: on 23 November 1984, a Friday (the day of the week traditionally set aside for matters of only minor importance), an open debate was held in the House of Commons to test elected representatives' reactions to the Warnock Report.

I attended Parliament myself that day, in the visitors' gallery. The debate had been publicised well in advance, and the House was very well attended. The opponents of Warnock came in force, hoping to repeat their recent success in the Lords.

The Government opened the debate. Uneasily aware of the massed critics waiting to pounce, the Minister of State tried to be all things to all people. He accepted the intensity of public feeling: help for the infertile was desirable, but so were controls. The important thing was to remain open-minded about future advances. Commercial surrogacy was probably a bad thing; he agreed with Warnock that children conceived by donor insemination should be legitimised and that everything possible should be done to eliminate genetic diseases; but on the 14-day limit for embryo research he was less certain, and took notice of the fact that even the Church of England was divided on the matter.

It was a speech that discreetly opened the way for the supporters of Warnock. Michael Meacher, who had been MP for Oldham at the time when Louise Brown was born there, was understandably sympathetic: he recognised that his was the first generation ever to have such a pressing need to answer the question 'what is the nature and status of a human being?', but he felt that science and medicine should be given every possible opportunity to develop freely. Leo Abse, too, was an eloquent supporter. He openly celebrated in-vitro fertilisation, criticised the Medical Research Council for failing to support Oldham's pioneering work, and argued strongly that the implications of embryo research were too broad for any stance against them to be taken from a narrowly moral, historical position. He commented unfavourably on the Church's attitudes, the Virgin Birth, and reminded members of the affair between Galileo and the Pope.

Warnock had supporters among the assembled MPs, several of them women who spoke with particular conviction. But by now Warnock's opponents were getting restless. Among the first to catch the Speaker's eyes was Sir Bernard Braine.

Sir Bernard was robust in his denunciations. He found absolutely no trace of guiding moral principles in the Warnock Report. He was shocked at its complaisance, at its willingness to allow embryos to be experimented upon, mutilated, frozen for as long as ten years and then simply killed. The lack in it of any defence of marriage as the proper framework in which to raise children offended him deeply. And the need for embryo research was greatly overstated: he himself had spoken to Jerome Lejeune, the discoverer of Down's syndrome, and had been told that no embryo research was needed in order to cure it.

He spoke powerfully. 'I have been privileged to be a Member for almost thirty-five years, and never in all that time have I approached any subject with a greater sense of fear than this . . .' He went on to quote Jeremiah: 'Before I formed thee in the belly I knew thee; and before thou cometh forth out of the womb I sanctified thee.'

'How can any civilised society,' he asked, 'accept that on the thirteenth day the embryo does not count, it is just a piece of jelly; but at one minute past midnight on the fourteenth day it suddenly becomes a human person who is entitled to the full protection of the law?'

(I agreed with him, incidentally, in finding this judgment of Warnock curiously anomalous — but unfortunately from the diametrically opposite standpoint!)

After Sir Bernard, as in the House of Lords, once again the flood-gates of reactionary opinion were opened. The Reverend Ian Paisley, a Protestant leader from Northern Ireland and a fervent believer in the Virgin Birth, had no doubt at all that conception, life, the formation of the body and birth itself were all mysterious and miraculous — and were therefore best left alone. For him, an embryo's right to life was of supreme importance — far more important than the right to have a family — and yet freezing was unacceptable . . . and furthermore, once scientists had been given fourteen days for their research they'd soon be back for more. He even found himself agreeing with John Hume, a Roman Catholic also from Northern Ireland, for the very first time since they had joined Parliament together.

The opponents of Warnock were vociferous to the end. Mrs Peacock believed that the freezing of embryos must erode established moral standards, and called for a ban on in-vitro fertilisation except between husband and wife. The recurrent claim was that an embryo was 'a human being with a potential for full human development', and many MPs — Sir Hugh Rossi in particular — demanded far stricter rules than Warnock's.

No vote had been intended, and none was taken. But the majority against in-vitro fertilisation and everything to do with it was obvious. The debate was a disaster for the Warnock Report, and, following its fate now in both Lords and Commons, its future looked highly unpromising.

Further political moves were inevitable. Knowing that they were on top, the opposition were impatient, eager to finish off Warnock once and for all. For a short time they lacked a leader, but then one emerged: Mr Enoch Powell. He was a brilliant speaker and a formidable parliamentarian, an ex-minister for the Conservatives and now an MP for Northern Ireland, and he went on record as finding the Warnock Report repugnant. His belief in and respect for life prevented him from accepting embryo research, and he insisted on far tighter controls for in-vitro fertilisation than Warnock proposed.

Although a willing spokesman for the anti-Warnock movement, Mr Powell was without a platform in the House, since the government was pointedly biding its time and avoiding further parliamentary confrontation. But then, unexpectedly, Mr Powell's chance came.

Every year a small number of Private Members' Bills are put before the House of Commons, and a ballot is held among those members who have given notice that they hope to present some personal item of legislation. Mr Powell entered the ballot for 1985 and happened to be chosen, gaining fourth place. He immediately gathered a team of supporters, and together they composed a bill intended to control in-vitro fertilisation, which they called the Unborn Children (Protection) Bill.

It is curious, incidentally, that this title should have got past Mr Powell's sharp legal eye, for it seriously begged the question, containing as it did the so far unproved assumption that embryos were indeed already 'Unborn Children'. But worse was to follow:

UNBORN CHILDREN (PROTECTION) BILL.
Except with the authority of the Secretary of State under this Act, no person shall —
(a) procure the fertilisation of human ovum in vitro (that is to say, elsewhere than in the body of a woman) or
(b) have in his possession a human embryo produced by in-vitro fertilisation.

The Secretary of State's authority
(a)  shall be given expressly for the purpose of enabling a named woman to bear a child by means of embryo insertion, and not for any other purpose
(b)  shall be given in writing and only when applied for, in the prescribed form, by two registered medical practitioners, and
(c)  shall specify  (i) the person by whom, or under whose directions the procedure of in-vitro fertilisation and embryo insertion are authorised to be carried out
(ii) the place or places where any such procedure is to be carried out, and . . .

The provisions and prohibitions continued down many pages. Those in charge of embryos had to be named. The Secretary of State's authority lasted for four months and must then be renewed, but would lapse again when the embryo was replaced. And there were fines laid down, and imprisonment, should any of the terms be defied. The Bill was a legal maze, at every corner of which criminality lurked for the unwary. And its purpose, seemingly, was to stifle research and to deny in-vitro fertilisation to all but the very few women who passed its stringent — and always changeable — criteria.

Mr Powell's Bill opposed Warnock in a very fundamental sense: it allowed no middle way, no compromise between differing opinions and convictions, and it constituted a savage attack upon civil liberties. The requirement for all patients individually to gain the Secretary of State's consent before they conceived a child amounted to instituting a licence for procreation. It was a denial of every citizen's basic human rights and it was dangerously open to abuse. Untempered by any detectable human feeling, it was bad politics and also bad medicine.

Many people, like me, saw the Bill as misjudged and tyrannical. Certainly IVF and embryo research must be monitored, but not in this destructive fashion. Opposition to it mounted among members of the general public as well as politicians and lawyers, doctors and scientists. But Mr

Powell was excellently organised, and he and his supporters remained optimistic.

On 15 February 1985 Mr Powell's Bill came before the House for its second reading. Any public petitions to Parliament must be read before a debate begins and in this case there were many, all of them objecting to in-vitro fertilisation and research on embryos. The petition organised by LIFE now carried more than two million signatures, collected in under six months and representing a national record. If this was genuinely the feeling of the nation then the battle against the forces of reaction was already lost.

Mr Powell presented his Bill. 'This Bill has a single and simple purpose. It is to render it unlawful for a human embryo created by in-vitro fertilisation to be used as the subject of experiments, or indeed in any other way, or for any purpose except to enable a woman to bear a child . . .' Later, he said, 'When I first read the Warnock Report I had a sense of revulsion and repugnance . . .'

Several women MPs opposed him. Ms Richardson criticised every provision of his Bill: she stressed the need for controlled research and was angered that the civil liberties of the infertile might be infringed by the requirement for political consent in the matter of having a child: 'I prefer to take not just the emotive views of people, but the informed view, for example, of the National Federation of Women's Institutes . . . They reluctantly agree with the Warnock Committee that research on human embryos should be permitted . . . under licence, up to the fourteenth day after fertilisation.'

She was unsympathetic towards the moral arguments Mr Powell presented for the protection of embryos, since even he accepted IUDs as a contraceptive measure, and these expelled embryos from the womb with considerable efficiency. Another woman, Ms Short, agreed with her, criticising the wholesale nature of the petition and its vague terms, and demanding that women be given more rights in the making of decisions concerning reproduction.

Mr Meadowcroft opposed the Bill also. He was worried by the breadth of the powers it proposed giving to the Secretary of State, and by its insistence that all embryos be replaced in the mother (this last, in fact, had always made no medical sense at all). And Mr Abse spoke vehemently too, protesting against the Bill's reactionary nature, and its clear intention to suppress even the most responsible scientific research.

Inevitably Mr Powell had his supporters. Mrs Winterton quoted the Royal College of General Practitioners, which had asked for a moratorium on embryo research, and Mr St John Stevas quoted Aldous Huxley's vision of a brave new world in their support. Sir Bernard Braine had his quotation ready too: after raising the spectre of the Nazi concentration camps and the Nuremberg Trials, he quoted William Pitt: 'Necessity is the plea for every infringement of human freedom. It is the argument of tyrants. It is the creed of slaves.'

Two churchmen joined in, Martin Smith and Ian Paisley, both accusing scientists of wanting to play God, and insisting that the unborn child must not fall prey to their greed for knowledge and power. For another MP, Mr Pawsey, the status of life itself was under debate, now that science had abandoned all the teachings of the Church. Dr Bray was in a dilemma – he saw the need for research, but his conscience obliged him to support Mr Powell. Mr Beith had no such problem: he considered it an excellent thing that parents should be licensed to have children; he was a Liberal by profession!

The debate turned out to be a repeat of that in the Lords. A few MPs tried to stem the reactionary flood, pointing out that all the old arguments about playing God, and the Nazi concentration camps, and power-crazed scientists had been raised and dealt with years before, at the time of the original

Abortion Act, and that the present law, which allowed
fetuses to be destroyed up to the twenty-eighth week, had
been enormously beneficial in supporting research to help
the infertile and to diagnose genetic handicaps, but the
battle was lost. No one was listening.

The vote was taken, and Mr Powell's supporters won —
238 votes to 66. It was a resounding and, one might have
thought, a conclusive victory. But in fact that day we had
heard the emotions of the House speaking — its heart rather
than its head, and certainly not a wise combination of both
— and as the actual black-and-white provisions of Mr
Powell's Bill came to be rationally considered the need for
extensive amendment became blindingly obvious.

Meanwhile, many other European countries were showing no distaste at all for the Warnock Report. Belgium,
Sweden and Germany, in particular, welcomed it and
worked within its guidelines, and the European Parliament
accepted it as a basis for discussion. During 1985 debates on
the subject of embryo research took place in the parliaments
of six European countries, seemingly with none of the
rancorous hysteria seen in Britain.

Words of warning were spoken of course, and necessarily, but usually with the Cartesian objectivity of Madame
Questiaux, the French ex-Minister of Social Affairs, when
for example she addressed the Legal Commission of the
Parliament of Europe:

. . . the new techniques of artificial reproduction are not at all
rejected by public opinion. Perhaps I have misunderstood Lady
Warnock. But thus far I, at any rate, have not had any impression
of fear. On the contrary . . . it is the medical practitioners and
scientists who are saying to us 'Advise us, stop us from doing the
worst,' and . . . the public who is saying 'Go ahead,' as though in
this area human interference and science fiction were not
frightening. But it is also my impression that the people who are
so trustful of science have not really thought about the way in
which the act of reproduction is being sub-divided and broken
up.

Now, in Britain, Mr Powell's retrogressive Bill was due for its third reading. If it won, then it would go to the Lords, who would almost certainly support it. And then, after a final debate in the Commons, it would become law. But it needed considerable amendment before, in the cold, unemotional light of its third reading, it would gain a majority, and its opponents were working hard. Most of these amendments were blocked in committee as general enthusiasm waned, so that when it returned to the House little other than the clause on patient registration had in fact been changed.

Mr Powell fought on. He knew he was in trouble and he manoeuvred skilfully, but in the end enough opinion was against him, he faced a filibuster, and he ran out of time. He was unable to proceed and his Bill was lost – until some future session when someone else might revive it.

Significantly, this happened to be at roughly the time when an American commercial agency offering to organise surrogate mothers for childless couples became headline news in Britain. The public was outraged and a hue and cry developed, and the agency's client, Mrs Cotton, was hounded unmercifully by reporters as she delivered her baby and handed it over to the commissioning couple. The controversy shifted popular interest from Mr Powell's Bill to the question of commercial surrogacy and the government, relieved, stepped in with a bill it felt safer with.

On 7 March 1985, the Secretary of State, Mr Norman Fowler, rose again, now with the government's own Surrogacy Arrangements Bill: 'Over the last few months there has been increasing concern about the practice of surrogacy . . . in particular [about] the activities of agencies which operate to provide surrogacy arrangements on a commercial basis . . . The government believes that commercial surrogacy is in principle undesirable.'

He had accurately judged the mood of the House, and the nation. The will to take a firm stand, and quickly, was generally accepted, and if this required compromise, then so be it. Only one small area of disagreement arose. Ms Richardson supported the government view that only commercial surrogacy should be discussed, while Sir Hugh Rossi perceived an illogicality in this.

'If a human act is intrinsically good or bad,' he asked, 'how can the payment or non-payment for that act alter its essential nature? . . . If all surrogacy, commercial or non-commercial, were to be made illegal, would we not avoid a great many legal and sociological problems?'

He may well have been right. But a logical law is not always a good law, and neither is it always one capable of being enforced, and the House recognised that private, family-based surrogacy would continue to take place, no matter what. So the debate concentrated on commercial surrogacy and, in response to strong public sentiment, no time was wasted. The government's Bill was introduced, debated, passed, and it became law, all in just over three months. Thus, on 16 July 1985, Britain became the first country in the world to ban commercial surrogacy.

In the House of Lords some members had resisted, arguing for a ban on private as well as commercial surrogacy, enforceable or not, but they had been defeated. The Bishop of Ripon and other churchmen opposed them, broad-mindedly pointing out that private surrogacy might well constitute a loving act, a service generously provided between one woman and another.

In its final form the Bill was directed not against the commissioning parents or the surrogate mothers, but against agencies, their negotiators and advertisers. All their commercial activities were banned, and anyone breaching the law was liable to three months in prison. The Bill may have been hasty, but it met with widespread popular approval.

A year or so later Parliament might not have been able to take such a decisive step. With the acceptance by the states of Europe of the Single European Act, some of the two Houses' traditional authority had slipped away. As Lord

Denning put it in *The Times* for 3 November 1986, 'It creates a new legal order in international law, and also in our constitutional law. Parliamentary sovereignty has gone . . . Community law, as declared by the European Court, is superior over any act of our Parliament that is inconsistent with it.'

And indeed, in the matter of embryo research for one, the British Parliament's autonomy was never likely to be so complete. The Council of Europe was already busy, the Legal Affairs Committee of its Parliamentary Assembly having already issued a report containing its own recommendations. 'The Assembly . . . calls on the governments of the member states to . . . forbid any production of human embryos in vitro for the purpose of research during their life or after death . . . [and to] forbid the creation of identical human beings by cloning or other methods.'

Although rejecting the creation of research embryos, the committee proposed acceptance of the Warnock 14-day rule for research on embryos not specifically created for this purpose. But spare part surgery worried them, as did the use of fetal tissue to repair a ravaging illness in adult or child: 'It shall be forbidden to keep embryos or fetuses alive artificially for the purpose of removing usable material . . . The use of *dead* embryos or fetuses must be an exceptional measure, justified in the present state of knowledge, by the rare nature of the illness treated . . .' The Parliamentary Assembly began to debate its recommendations, facing almost insoluble differences of opinion among its member states.

In Britain, however, Mr Powell's supporters were not easily deterred. His Unborn Children (Protection) Bill was briefly revived twice in 1986 by Mr Hargreaves, and yet again in 1987 by Mr Burt. It was unsuccessful on these occasions, but its reappearance put pressure upon the government to make at least a show of doing something, and in November 1987 a consultative document was put before Parliament: Human Fertilisation and Embryology: A

Framework for Legislation. At that time legislation was promised within a year or so, perhaps after a general election.

In Australia, however, the Victorian State Legislature took decisive action, in the form of its Infertility (Medical Procedures) Act which was to be introduced in stages between 1985 and 1987. Many of the comments made by members during the debate were depressingly familiar.

The Hon. D.N. Evans reminded his fellow-members that, 'A number of wild claims have been made . . . brave new world theories, the possibility of a man-ape, things of that nature . . .' The Hon. G.P. Connard agreed with him: 'Cloning could be just around the corner. I suggest that honourable members would be horrified if forty-four Mr Connards debated the same measure!'

But once the jokes were over, the provisions of the Infertility (Medical Procedures) Act turned out to be fiercely reactionary and prohibitive. Fertilisation was judged to be the moment when human life began, and under the requirements of the Declaration of Helsinki on human rights, guardianship was mandatory from that moment on. Studies on embryos were restricted to 'therapeutic research' (whatever that may mean, since there is virtually no therapy anyone can offer a sick embryo), and their destruction was banned. A Standing Review and Advisory Committee was set up to approve procedures and assess penalties, as well as to designate those centres permitted to undertake in-vitro fertilisation and to name those doctors entitled to take part.

In Victoria, therefore, legislation promised not only to regulate in-vitro fertilisation and embryo research for the first time ever, but also to regulate it almost out of existence. The pioneering work being done there was brought to a halt, and the measures seemed set to spread to other Australian states.

In France, as we have already seen, the 1987 decisions of the National Ethical Committee were more liberal, but also more confused. Embryo research was permissible and the 14-day rule was judged to rest on no sound ethical or scientific basis — but then the committee proposed a seven-day rule instead. Also, each individual research project had to gain the committee's approval, and modifications in human genetics, the gestation of human embryos in animals, ecogenesis and parthenogenesis (none of which was being seriously studied) were all banned. Doubts were expressed about the holding of embryos in a deep freeze should their mother become pregnant with fresh embryos (a somewhat arcane circumstance), and techniques for identifying genetic disease in embryos (perhaps embryology's most exciting area of potential development) were severely restricted.

In Germany, too, although no actual legislation yet exists, the International Association of Penal Law, meeting in Freiberg in 1987, has issued some sweeping proposals. Among other matters, it recommends:

i.    The prohibition of embryos created for purposes other than human procreation.
ii.   The establishment of minimim standards of safeguard for gamete donation, in particular through an obligation to keep available information about donor characteristics that might be relevant to the health of the recipient and/or her offspring.
iii.  The prohibition of extra-corporeal cultivation of embryos beyond the development stage reached by natural nidation.
iv.   The prevention of any trade in embryos and of the commercialisation of pregnancies by so-called surrogate motherhood.
v.    That the inviolability of genetic inheritance against artificial intervention should be protected by law.
vi.   That the cloning of human beings should be made a criminal offence.
vii.  That all attempts to produce hybrids and chimaeras by means of karyogamy of human germ cells with those of animals should also be made criminal offences.

In the USA, however, an embryologist's life is probably even more difficult than it is in Europe. Admittedly the Supreme Court's long-standing ruling on abortion lays down twelve weeks as the moment when the mother's rights become paramount, and during the time before that the US Ethics Advisory Board has agreed 'that the human embryo is entitled to profound respect: but this respect does not necessarily encompass the full legal and moral rights attributed to persons.' But each American state has its own rules and laws, and state legislatures can make new laws at will, or arbitrarily apply existing regulations concerning foetuses to IVF and research on embryos. In some states they can compel a doctor to replace every successful IVF embryo, or, as in Illinois, make him the embryo's custodian and liable in criminal law for its life and health.

Here in Britain, meanwhile, an uneasy hiatus has descended. This is unsatisfactory since it leaves nothing decided and simply represents an opting out on the part of both government and society at large. Tacit acceptance of the Warnock Report is the order of the day. The Conservatives' 1987 consultative document promised a licensing authority with broad powers backed by harsh legal penalties.

The Chairman must be . . . neither a qualified medical practitioner nor a scientist involved in work using human gametes or embryos . . . At least half the members should be lay, and at least one-third doctors or scientists . . . The Statutory Licensing Authority will have a duty to draw up a Code of Practice . . . which might include guidelines for screening of donors; obtaining consent from patients and donors; use of stored gametes and embryos; counselling; and appropriate training and experience for medical and nursing staff . . . It will be a criminal offence to bring into existence, use or store a human embryo outside the body without an appropriate licence . . . to use gametes donated by a third party . . . to furnish false or misleading information for the purpose of . . . assisting another person in obtaining a licence . . .

MPs would have the choice over embryo research, Warnock or Powell. As yet nothing has come of these recommendations. And with luck nothing will come of them, for it is my belief, as I wrote with an American lawyer, Dave Sharpe, back in 1971, that 'what is needed is not heavy-handed statute . . . but a simple organisation, easily approached and consulted. Advisers are needed whose achievements and attitudes make them worth listening to . . . The stress would be on individual and private action, inquiry and consultation, not on authority, control bureaucracy, or laws with teeth.'

In any case, rumours abound that no bill will come in the near future. Maybe the Government's legislation programme genuinely is too full. More to the point, perhaps, are the fears that any bill would be hijacked by MPs wishing simply to curb abortion and embryo research.

Meanwhile, however, legislation is passed elsewhere. South Australia penalises surrogacy, has established an advisory council, and insists that research on embryos ends 'at the point where implantation would normally occur' provided it is not detrimental to an embryo. Queensland proposes to ban surrogacy and France's supreme court has presented new regulations to the government. The words of Madam Questiaux sum up much of the political uncertainty.

A law is needed, why? First of all, because a conflict on principle exists . . . On the one hand, the idea is strongly spread by our Anglo-Saxon friends that people have the right to dispose of themselves, their families and embryos that could be conceived from them . . . But faced with this in our country . . . no general principle exists to say that a person has [such a] right . . . The jurist will not need to struggle with problems over scientific definitions of the embryo . . . it is highly probable that neither our society, nor many others, will accept the idea that one may produce embryos simply for research . . . Juridical circles must [find] formulas that reconcile scientific evaluations with the ethical viewpoint [and] must learn not to be too pretentious . . . not lay down things in laws too soon . . .

# 11
# Conclusions

Flourishing scientific research is certain to tax the moral attitudes of society. Today, more than ever before, science probes deeply into every aspect of human life, examining and redefining literally everything in the universe, from the very beginnings of matter, the emergence of life, to the end of all things and the nature of death itself. Today, more than ever before, we must listen and look, and question, always responding imaginatively to the discoveries and demands of new disciplines.

The philosophy of science appeals to me particularly perhaps because I am myself a scientist. For this reason, Sir Karl Popper makes an especial impact on me, for he puts into words the emotions and outlook I feel:

'Science is most significant as one of the greatest spiritual adventures that man has yet known,' he wrote. '[Its] theories are not bodies of impersonal facts about the world but are products of the human mind . . . personal achievements of an astonishing order. Theories arise . . . in dreams or dreamlike states: in flashes of inspiration . . . all organisms are constantly, day and night, engaged in problem solving . . .'

The great theories of science fill me with wonder. Jacques Monod, a French philosopher of science, places man in perspective in a huge impersonal universe, exposed, as are all animals, to blind evolutionary pressures: 'he lives on the boundary of an alien world; a world deaf to his music and as indifferent to his hopes as it is to his sufferings or his crimes.' Astronomers join in this interpretation of man's condition. Read the words of one of them, Martin Rees: 'All the common elements . . . of which we are made, were built up from primordial hydrogen and helium by nuclear transmutations inside stars which exploded before our solar system was formed. We are literally made from the ashes of long-dead stars.' Julian Huxley, a British philosopher of science, gives the same message as Popper, but less starkly: 'Scientific integration has now for the first time begun to cover the entire range of phenomena involved in human destiny and . . . [is] being forced to deal with the phenomena of values.'

Concepts such as evolution, thermodynamics, DNA raise a sense of wonder but also a sense of reality. How can any scientist be other than religious as he uncovers this ordered beauty? Not religious in the Church's sense, perhaps, but certainly in his own. And all these marvellous but uncomfortable facts about our origins or our destiny have to be built into a system of values. Scientific facts are always open to change, for we know all too well the transitional nature of many scientific theories, and this knowledge makes me distrust easy answers, certainty, completeness, finality, absolutism. These seem to me to be shelters for those seeking emotional or intellectual comfort, and empty promises for those unprepared to consider the facts of life as they are.

Many non-scientists see a more limited role for science, almost a fact-gathering exercise providing neither values, morals, nor standards. I suppose those suspicious of the mysterious, awe-inspiring concepts of science may prefer to believe in the interpretation offered by the Vatican's Congregation for the Doctrine of the Faith: 'Thus, science and technology require, for their own intrinsic meaning, an unconditional respect for the fundamental criteria of the moral law; that is to say, they must both be at the service of the human person, of his inalienable rights, and of his true and integral good . . . No biologist or doctor can reasonably claim, by virtue of his scientific competence, to be able to decide on people's origin and destiny.' Or, as expressed more simply by a *Times* correspondent (18 April 1987), science's 'empirical scepticism' has 'invaded moral consciousness and is at the root of the contemporary crisis of faith. It asserts that what is not provable is not knowable.'

My answer to the Vatican is that moral laws must be based on what man knows about himself, and that this knowledge inevitably comes largely from science. As the physicist Jacob Bronowski pointed out, 'What makes the biological machinery of man so powerful is that it modifies his actions through his imagination: it makes him able to symbolise, to project himself into the consequences of his acts, to conceptualise his plans, and to weigh them one against another as a system of values . . .' Julian Huxley agreed: 'Today the God hypothesis has ceased to be scientifically tenable, has lost its explanatory value and is becoming an intellectual burden to our thought . . .'

Scientists should be wary, however: so much remains unexplained, mysterious — particularly the ways in which we function in making judgments, in our humour, in our standards — even in our love. Pair-bonding, as the behaviourists call it, is one thing; love, as you and I know it, is surely quite another. Scientists are not always humble either, for some physicists predict a 'theory of everything' and molecular biologists propose to reduce man to his atoms as a way to understand him better, and even plan to modify him one day. The latter have been sharply rebuked by Mary Midgley, a tireless philosopher stalking their every word, their every claim:

'The discovery of DNA [has] combined with a sense of commanding position on the frontiers of the physical and biological sciences . . . [so that molecular biologists] appear to be . . . missionaries . . . spreading physical methods over all . . . remaining intellectual areas of the slightest interest.'

My own interest in systems of values began thirty years ago as a PhD student in Edinburgh, and grew strongly in Oldham, when Patrick, Jean and I researched the mysteries of human conception. More than any other scientific study I had done, ripening human eggs in vitro, fertilising them and growing them as embryos, all this forced me to wonder about their rights and the rights of patients, to make decisions about my own ethics, and then to try to convince other members of society that my position was reasonable and, in Socrates' sense, virtuous. Those debates have extended to an unbelievable breadth of society since then, yet I still wonder if any of us have had our minds changed over all these years. One thing, though, must be clear to everyone. Human reproduction has always raised matters of intense ethical concern, and will continue to do so.

Encouragingly, the moral debate about embryos has embraced people in all walks of life, politicians, churchmen, philosophers, scientists and ordinary men and women. Even so, decisions of enormous ethical implications have been made almost without question, though widely reported by the world's press. Sometimes they are made by governments, sometimes by ethical or professional organisations, and occasionally by individuals. Take population policies, for example. Several countries have decided to cajole their people into producing more or fewer children simply by using their political power, irrespective of individual need. Malaysia has decided to increase its population fivefold, from fourteen million to seventy million, in order to become a dynamic force in Southeast Asia. Its neighbour, Singapore, tries to encourage more births also, fearful because its women have only 1.4 children each. It wants more intelligent children too, so its cleverer citizens will be especially helped to produce more. Quebec wants more French speakers to counter the English-speaking tide. Eastern European countries repeal abortion laws to stimulate the population growth, and even Western countries, such as Germany, bribe their womenfolk to become more fertile. On the other hand, the perils of China's one-child population policy are well known, the general disobedience and the infanticide of girls, so that now the Government promises to let rural couples have a second child if their first baby is a girl.

Sometimes, too, courts of law make decisions of immense ethical importance. The US Supreme Court handed down a historic decision, *Roe* v *Wade*, in 1973, giving American women the right to decide on abortion in the first third of pregnancy, granting a balance between her and her fetus's rights in the second third of pregnancy, and giving the fetus major rights in the final third. This has become the fundamental abortion law of the USA, despite the opposition of Catholics and others who do their best to overturn it.

Then there are the non-political or non-judicial organisations, pressure groups such as LIFE, Friends of the Earth, even some professional organisations, that campaign over abortion, environmental pollution, the rights of animals, and become powerful, respected, their ethical standards widely accepted.

Finally, there is the brave individual who embarks on a crusade, determined to prove to the world that things are not what they should be. Such people often fight single-handed against immense odds as they present new ideas, new possibilities for the public to accept or reject. The British doctor, Dr Bourne, aborted a girl who had been raped, after telling the police of his intention: he was duly charged, tried and acquitted and so brought about new abortion laws in Britain. He made his own decision, then convinced others. Margaret Sanger did a similar job over contraception for the masses in New York. Mother Theresa does the same for the world's poor. And, twenty years ago, three people in Oldham revolutionised human conception, determined to help a previously neglected group of people. Sadly, I am our little group's only survivor.

Two of the team are now dead. Jean Purdy, the patient, indomitable helper without whom none of our work would have been possible, died in 1985. She was not yet forty when a small black wart erupted, an incurable melanoma, which quickly spread its cancerous cells throughout her body.

And then, in 1988, Patrick Steptoe was killed by cancer also. One day, very possibly, the lives of patients like him and Jean Purdy will be saved by precisely the lines of research into early embryology that they themselves pioneered. I watched Patrick in his final months and wished with all my heart that for him and for so many others the cure could have come sooner. He was still at work, battling on against his pain and debilitation, fighting his disease with all the techniques medicine had to offer, and with a spirit that, as always, refused to give in. I watched him at Bourn Hall with the children and grateful parents who return there, a frail old man, grey with suffering as he stooped to talk and laugh with them. For myself, I judge all doctors by my knowledge of Patrick, and I hope that each one of those children may remember him, and understand his courage and his love.

Few doctors have achieved what he did. He pioneered two techniques, laparoscopy and IVF, defended IVF against the law and the bigots, and saw it spread worldwide in his lifetime. He lived to know that somewhere in the world more than one thousand Bourn Hall babies, conceived in vitro, were growing up beloved, normal, and in good health. And he lived to see his work legitimised and respected around the world.

As for me, it was a practical, scientific outlook that drove me on, convinced we were right to employ our skills as we did. IVF, surrogacy, genetic screening, stem cells, all these offer hope to thousands upon thousands of people. And now, writing out of all this experience in December 1988, how do I see the results of all our work? Has all the effort been worth it? Where do we stand, in the last part of the twentieth century, in relation to scientific advances, the ethical upheavals, the new medical understanding that has emerged from those long years of struggle?

It has certainly been worth it, for some things have been

permanently changed for the better. IVF is accepted worldwide for the alleviation of infertility, and will never be outlawed now. Improvements are certainly needed, in particular to help the spermatozoa of men with a low or abnormal sperm count to penetrate egg membrane which in some cases bars fertilisation, but people of every race and religion all over the world have benefitted from IVF. Soon, one in every two hundred French babies might be conceived this way.

The effort has been worth it in another sense. In-vitro fertilisation, donor insemination, frozen embryos, embryo accepted guidelines, and the ethical revolution has matched the scientific and medical revolution. In Britain, there is still no legislation, but the guidelines proposed by the Warnock Report have been adopted by a new Voluntary Licensing Authority (VLA), an unofficial watchdog over the affairs of assisted conception. Any guidelines are better than none in this litigious and accusatory world, if only to protect scientists like me from the risk of being labelled as immoral or put on trial as criminals or murderers. In America, the National Commission for the Protection of Human Subjects of Biomedical and Behavioural Research has guidelines demanding prior studies on animals and non-pregnant humans, and insisting that the new knowledge being sought must satisfy certain criteria of worth and importance. The risks and benefits to mother and fetus must have been evaluated, informed consent sought and granted, and subjects selected to ensure that risks and benefits do not fall inequitably among economic, racial, ethnic and social classes. And in France the National Ethical Committee advises its government, keeping one watchful eye on new developments and another on public reactions to them.

In many ways, sadly, the British Voluntary Licensing Authority is an unfortunate creation, a curious union between the democratic Royal College of Obstetricians and the unelected Medical Research Council — which incidentally has for some years been funding and carrying out embryo research in its own laboratories, including the creation of research embryos by the hundred, which activities should have prohibited it from ever having any ethical authority whatsoever. Nevertheless, the VLA issued its judgments: no cloning, hybrids or human babies in animals were allowed, even though no one was attempting them anyway. Then it supported the Warnock 14-day rule, and announced that before day 14, the embryo we had all been studying was actually a 'pre-embryo'.

Predictably, the ethicists were scathing. 'A Humpty-Dumpty word . . . to diminish the status of the newly-conceived embryo in the eye of the public,' commented Ken Hargreaves MP as he reintroduced his own Humpty-Dumpty measure, the Unborn Children Bill, in the House of Commons. 'Manipulating words to polarise ethical discussions,' decided David Davies, a member of the Warnock Committee. 'Behaviour-gathering terms rather than apparently descriptive terms,' concluded Margaret Sommerville in evidence to the Victorian Senate, in Australia.

Why did the VLA choose such a term as 'pre-embryo'? It evidently wanted to differentiate between the embryo and the placenta, which forms over a similar period of days. They pointed out that before this time there is no certainty which cells are embryonic and which placental, although these tissues actually separate on day 9 and not day 14. Perhaps they also felt that this lack of certainty gave more ethical justification for research. But the placenta is, in any case, a fundamental organ of the embryo, functioning as its lungs, food supply, gas supply, a cushion against shock and any immunological attack from its mother and many others. But 'pre-embryo' remains a weasel word to have chosen, particularly in the middle of an important ethical argument.

The VLA also supported the 14-day rule about embryo research. They may have done so because they felt public opinion could just about accept this period, if it could be justified, whereas any extension would have been rejected. In fact there is no clear scientific or medical reason for choosing day 14 rather than day 12 or day 18: as a time limit it is entirely arbitrary, no stronger ethically or medically than any other. The so-called 'primitive streak' which has appeared by then is merely a band of migrating cells that seed or form many organs of the body. Certainly when it has appeared there is no longer any doubt where the head and tail of the embryo will lie, or where its left and right sides will be, but many other equally significant tissues have appeared earlier — the placenta, brain and blood — and many will appear later. The large forebrain, characteristic of higher mammals, doesn't show strongly until day 30, when the rudiments also appear of the first sense organ, the eye. And although separate twins cannot arise after day 14, conjoined twins can apparently be formed afterwards, and can result in two distinct people. Conjoined twins in the USA have lived, worked, married and fathered children, taking turns to live in their respective homes, and surviving happily to a ripe old age.

In the final analysis, individual doctors or scientists have to make up their own minds about their ethical stance, just as we had to so many years ago. They have to face the arguments, whether life is an endless thread, or has an instant, off/on beginning. They have to decide what is alive — embryos, fetuses and children (and so too spermatozoa and unfertilised eggs?) — and to decide further which groups should be given absolute protection or if a claim to *potential* humanity is by implication a denial of *present* humanity, which gets nobody anywhere. I myself believe human spermatozoa are just that — human — and so are human unfertilised eggs. And both should be protected particularly watchfully since humanity itself could become perverted if genetic engineers were recklessly to introduce new genes into them.

All those individuals now doing IVF must also decide if the day 14 rule is significant or not. For me, there has been and still is only one reasonable way in which to look at the rights of human embryos. They must grow as the embryo grows, reflecting its increasing complexity of tissues and details of organisation. Day 14 is a good general rule, but there must be exceptions when fundamental studies can be done only after this time. Anyone wishing to study an embryo, to use its tissues or destroy it, must find greater justification as it grows older. This is the gradualist approach, placing the onus on the researcher, on those who ultimately will make the day-to-day decisions. This proposal will shock absolutists, but not those doctors who already do society's bidding by aborting healthy months-old fetuses, or those scientists who then use those fetuses' tissues to mankind's benefit, making new medicines or better grafts.

Researching the causes of chromosomal diseases like Down's syndrome can be largely carried out before day 5. Discoveries about new contraceptive methods and some causes of infertility will arise from studies on the placenta, which forms between days 8–10. Neurobiologists research-ing the brain and its anomalies cannot begin until day 12 while cardiologists researching the development of the heart must wait for day 18. Most studies in vitro can be completed by day 25, and after that the current rules for using tissues from aborted foetuses will suffice. So the time of research in dispute is really very small indeed. It might be even smaller still, if the new drug RU486 is used for abortion, because embryonic tissue will become available at 18 or 20 days of gestation.

But for the moment the 14-day limit is what we have, and much research can be done within it. It does result, however, in the unreasonable possibility that a life-saving piece of research may suddenly, at one minute past midnight (on the fourteenth day?), become a criminal act, and an act, furthermore, that is criminal even though performed upon a microscopic entity, while the tissues of aborted fully-formed three- and four-months old fetuses may be legally experimented upon virtually without limit. I'm not neces-sarily arguing for a change in the law concerning research on abortuses, merely that logic should be applied to the legislation as a whole.

The VLA also accepted embryos created specifically for research, perhaps the only ethical authority in the world to do so. Ironically, I have reservations on this issue and have to move here into the notoriously difficult philosophical area of *intention*. I have no objection to research carried out upon abnormal embryos, embryos created for implantation and then, because their initial growth was not successful, never used for this purpose. Neither do I question work performed on frozen embryos no longer needed by their parents: they were also created with the intention of implantation, but their parents no longer want them so in a sense have aborted them. Their use for research satisfies the same ethical criteria as the use of abortuses from spontaneous or induced abortions. But the knowing creation of research embryos, their fate decided before they are conceived — simply to have three or four days of life, perhaps exposed to radioactive tracers or some other chemical — seems to me a very different, and significant step for a scientist to take. The decision to permit research embryos should be taken by politicians, not by scientists or doctors in their laboratories or clinics.

Back in 1975 I addressed the World Council of Churches on the subject, and I haven't changed my views since:

Some laboratories . . . accept the view that human embryos can be deliberately initiated in the laboratory and then destroyed later. This situation is very different from that occurring in clinical studies where the embryos have been created in attempts to cure infertility, and it cannot be justified by reference to current social practices where embryos or foetuses conceived accidentally are aborted by, for example, the use of the IUD or menstrual aspiration for birth control. Accepting fertilisation in vitro as a laboratory study in its own right can thus lead to the establishment of new values about early human growth . . .

Inevitably many of my colleagues disagree with me. Even our terminology can differ. As the biologist Anne

McLaren points out, writing in favour of research embryos, 'Embryo is an ambiguous term. What actually happens is that women who come in for sterilisation . . . are asked . . . to donate oöcytes for research purposes . . . This rings true to me. It's the end of one's own reproductive life and all those eggs in one's ovaries are going to waste. If they can be used to help . . . prevent genetic defects, that is an act of generosity.'

But I stand by the ethics of intention. In this at least, a theologian, Anthony Dyson, is on my side: 'In ethics one is concerned with intention, with the nature of an act, and with its consequences. Clearly, using an embryo . . . produced with a therapeutic intention could be argued to be different from creating one for specific research purposes . . . The importance of intention cannot be overestimated.'

The VLA should investigate research on 'spare' embryos in clinics that cannot establish – or do not wish to install – a freezing programme. Doctors in such clinics simply replace three or four – sometimes more – embryos, then use all the rest for research, being unable to freeze them for their patients' later benefit. If they can afford research, they should be able to afford the cost of freezing. The embryos are not theirs: they belong to the parents, and every attempt should be made to implant them.

The VLA apart, in Europe the French National Ethical Committee seems to live in its own sort of uncertainty. It does not accept the term 'pre-embryo', and like all the other committees it bans cloning, hybrids, and growing human embryos in animals. But then it makes a series of recommendations which seem to stand common sense on its head. It recognises human embryos as potential persons, but decides to permit research on them. It is uncertain if a mother should be allowed to keep deep-frozen embryos for a second pregnancy if she conceives the first time round with her fresh embryos. It disapproves of the day-14 rule about research on embryos – the first ethical committee to dismiss Warnock's ideas – because there are no ethical or scientific reasons for choosing such a particular day, but it then recommends that research should be limited to day 7 instead!

The muddle grows even worse. The Committee has decided to ban for three years all work on diagnosing inherited defects in human embryos growing in vitro. One reason for their decision is that replacing embryos found to be free from genetic defects paves the way for the selection of children by reference to their future qualities; an embryo should be respected for what it is, and the choice of which will live should not be decided by the manipulator (see J.P. Renard, *Human Reproduction*, in press). Also, these methods would be no substitute for the tried and tested prenatal diagnosis at ten or eighteen weeks of gestation.

This really is standing reason on its head. The Committee fails to distinguish the difference between negative eugenics, avoiding the birth of children with defects, and positive eugenics, making children superior by changing their characteristics in ways judged to be advantageous. There is all the difference in the world between these two techniques — one is defensive, the other offensive. Those embryos the French Committee will not diagnose at three or five days may well have to be aborted at three or six months, so the ban does no service to the embryo or the parents.

Even more surprising, this view is also advanced by Jacques Testart, the French introducer of propanediol for freezing human embryos:

Personally, I am against the genetic sorting of embryos, because it has created the illusion of the perfect child . . . An analogy with prenatal diagnosis cannot be made, because when it is known that a child bears a genetic anomaly, it remains a trial for the couple to endure, and in particular for the woman, the trial of abortion which is never a pleasure party. In the case of embryo sorting, leading to an in-vitro abortion, there is nothing left. 'Madame, you have seven embryos, there are three like this and four like that . . .' there is nothing left but to make a choice. So I believe that the method runs the risk ... of leading to an aberration of demand and recruitment.

Sometimes national committees must challenge individual doctors or clinics over the ethics of in-vitro fertilisation. Some of them replace ten or twelve or even more embryos in their patient in order to improve her chance of a pregnancy, knowing they may later have to 'cull' some of the resulting fetuses. They first talk her into accepting so many embryos, which cannot be easy, then they may have to persuade her to have several of the many fetuses she is carrying destroyed — simply to avoid the obstetric risks they themselves have created. Both patients and fetuses are devalued by exposing them to such risks. The doctors also lose ethical control of the situation, for if their patients refuse to have their fetuses culled, the doctors could face the clinical problems of a potentially disastrous multiple pregnancy.

The VLA, to its credit, has objected to the replacement of so many eggs or embryos, and had compelled one particular clinic to restrict its replacements to three of four.

Another difficult issue concerns donation: should a sister donate an oöcyte to a sister or should absolutely all donations be anonymous? Many doctors accept sister donations if counselling is done carefully: others feel a child might become attached to the donor if it discovered the truth of its parentage. Donors and recipients are probably equally divided in their views, so this is clearly not a case for hard and fast rules, yet the VLA chose to object to sister donation, and pressured a London clinic to abandon it. I believe the choice should be left to the patients, provided they are fully counselled.

It is also fascinating for me to watch as advances in IVF and its applications continue, some small, some large. An American company making IUDs and being sued for damages has offered to pay some of the women claimants suffering from infertility caused by infection to have a try for a child by IVF. And on the technical front, Swedish, Danish and Austrian doctors have improved ultrasound to such an extent that the collection of oöcytes is reduced to a fairly minor procedure, and laparoscopy has become rare. The simple means of collecting oöcytes, allied to the ease of replacing embryos, even threatens to displace GIFT.

Swedish and Mexican work on brain transplants has had an unexpected sequel. In Birmingham, here in Britain, Professor Hitchcock decided to repeat it. Tissues from aborted fetuses were injected into the brains of patients with Huntingdon's disease, hoping to control and even ameliorate their conditions. Professor Hitchcock believes this to be ethically acceptable even though he would never consider using tissues from embryos raised in vitro. 'The products of pregnancy have been collected routinely for many years for research,' he said recently. 'The tissue I used was collected routinely. It was not obtained specially for me. I do not know what method was used but it was obtained in the usual way. I have no connection with the surgeons who carried out the abortion.'

So fears instantly arose of a trade in fetuses, of a fetal tissue industry for the vast numbers of elderly people with brain disease, of mothers paid or pressured to conceive for organ banks, and the US National Institute of Health decided to suspend all federal funding for fetal tissue research. The British Medical Association, meanwhile, approved the transplants – under the conditions of the 1972 Peel Report which rules that transplant surgeons must not interfere with the mother's decision to abort, or with the abortion itself – but considered it unethical for a woman to become pregnant or to have an abortion solely to produce fetal material. A reasonable guideline, certainly, if difficult to administer.

Monsieur Byk, a French magistrate, lists topical items of interest he discovered for his 'Biomedical Ethics Newsletter' during the last six months of 1987. An Italian girl with leukemia received a marrow transplant from her 17-month-old brother conceived for the purpose. American and British research teams cloned calves using nuclei from 16-cell bovine embryos. An AIDS baby was born to a surrogate mother and no one wanted it, and three French courts struck down surrogate contracts because they contravened the inalienability of the human body. The staff of the Gynecological–Obstetrical Department in the Hôpital Catholique de Notre Dame de Bon-Secours in Paris resigned in protest because their IVF programme had been stopped in compliance with the Vatican's commendations, and an Appeal Court in Toulouse permitted the male companion of a woman inseminated with donor semen (not his) to cancel his acknowledgment of paternity even though he had concurred with the insemination.

Not surprisingly, developments in embryo research, embryonic grafts and genetic engineering have persuaded many countries to press ahead with proposed legislation. In Australia the State of Victoria has actually legislated, banning cloning, the making of hybrids and gestating human beings in animals, has restricted studies on embryos to 'therapeutic research' whatever that means, and their laws also prevent typing embryos for inherited disease.

Those Victorian Senators face a serious problem. Do they let women wear intrauterine devices or use post-coital contraceptives that expel embryos from their mother's womb or permit abortion to destroy fully-formed fetuses? If they permit any of these things, how can they reasonably pass laws to protect microscopic embryos in vitro? And how do they comfort parents fearing a handicapped child yet sick at the thought of aborting their fetus, when embryo research could offer a better alternative. They seem to be on the defensive, for one ethical committee there has now given consent to type embryos for inherited diseases.

The politicians of New South Wales, unimpressed by their Victorian counterparts, have passed more liberal laws about embryo research, possibly encouraging many a Victorian scientist to move to Sydney, for the more cordial atmosphere there. And in Germany an Embryo Bill, virtually preventing any embryo research, was withdrawn, perhaps for the technical reason that it was infringing individual German states' rights in such matters, or perhaps because the authorities had suddenly realised they were paying out money for contraception and abortion, but none for the alleviation of infertility.

And Britain? It was said that legislation would be definitely placed before Parliament within eighteen months according to Lord Skelmersdale, a Government Minister. Or would it? Rumours soon began to fly that legislation would not be introduced in 1988 after all, as I have described earlier, and some politicians now think about reintroducing Mr Powell's Bill. Decisions here about IVF, embryo research, surrogacy seem as far away as ever. Scientists will simply have to soldier on, protected only by their own ethical committees.

Middle ground is needed. The absolutists will never willingly give an inch, and neither will certain particularly determined research scientists. But the moment of fertilisation genuinely does not exist, and even if it did, it would not instantly confer upon the resulting embryo the same status as that of a newborn child. The gradualist approach is in fact already with us, as is demonstrated in the abortion issue, for even as I write this, the judgments of the US Supreme Court are being overtaken, as some doctors legally abort 24-week-old fetuses, while developments in neonatal care enable other doctors to save such premature babies.

Abortion, surrogate motherhood, in-vitro fertilisation, frozen embryos, embryo research — the issues they raise may be of differing ethical intensity, but they all make us uneasy and they all require us to take informed decisions ... and, characteristically, all we've produced so far is acrimony, arguments, amendments, confusion. And meanwhile, also characteristically, our unease deepens. The circle is vicious, and it must be broken. Shutting such questions away, not thinking about them, simply will not work. At some very deep level, people need to be happy with their society, to understand its decisions and approve.

Amidst all this ethical discussion, times were changing in

Bourn Hall. The death of Patrick Steptoe had been bad news, terrible news, and a wider base was needed to continue the work there. Out of the blue, in early 1988 at a particularly difficult time, an offer arrived to join up with the Hallam Clinic in London and with Aeres Serono, an international company with many interests. The new unit, Bourn Hallam, would be the largest in the world. On Monday 25 July 1988 – Louise Brown's tenth birthday – a headline appeared in the *Cambridge Evening News*: 'Swiss buy up test tube baby clinic'. The Medical Director would be Bridgett Mason, a doctor who years ago gave me advice which helped immeasurably with the conception of Louise Brown.

Yet ethical considerations must have the last word, as spoken by Sir Karl Popper, now a spry 86-year-old according to *The Times*, as he addressed the World Congress of Philosophy in August, 1988: 'As a scientific philosopher, Sir Karl has raised science almost to the level of art,' the paper claimed. He certainly had. 'The world . . . can now be seen to be . . . unfolding new possibilities,' he said. 'The propensity to survive for another year, or for twenty years, is not a property of man, but it is inherent in his situation . . . Next to music and art, science is the greatest, most beautiful, and most enlightening achievement of the human spirit. I abhor the noisy intellectual fashion that tries to denigrate science . . . I admire beyond anything the marvellous results achieved by the work of biologists and biochemists and made available through medicine to sufferers all over our beautiful earth.'

# Index